# The Mental Health Needs
and Young People

C000235867

# The Mental Health Needs of Children and Young People

## Guiding you to key issues and practices in CAMHS

Jane Padmore

Open University Press

Open University Press
McGraw-Hill Education
McGraw-Hill House
Shoppenhangers Road
Maidenhead
Berkshire
England
SL6 2QL

email: enquiries@openup.co.uk
world wide web: www.openup.co.uk

and Two Penn Plaza, New York, NY 10121-2289, USA


First published 2016

A catalogue record of this book is available from the British Library

ISBN-13: 978-0-33-526390-5
ISBN-10: 0-33-526390-9
eISBN: 978-0-33-526391-2

Library of Congress Cataloging-in-Publication Data
CIP data applied for

Typeset by Transforma Pvt. Ltd., Chennai, India
Printed and bound by CPI Group (UK) Ltd, Croydon, CR0 4YY

This book is about childhood and mental health. Many people have had a significant impact on my life, both as I was growing up and now, and the lives of my children. In recognition of this, I dedicate this book to my family.

To my husband, Roger, for his love, patience, support, and enduring belief in me.

To Ella and Luke for the fun, joy, and love they bring to my life.

To Naomi and Natalie, who have developed into wonderful women.

To my parents, Ian and Lesley, who gave me a childhood that ensured I have the resilience to face life and live it to the full.

To my sisters, Sally and Anna, not always together but always there for me.

To my uncle, David, for all the time, energy, and love he has given to the family.

To my aunt, Pam, for being there for my mother throughout.

To my grandparents, Alec, Jessie, Norman and Sheila, so many memories and they will never be forgotten.

To my mother-in-law, Vilma, the best mother-in-law a woman could have!

With special thanks to Rachel Crookes for her help in developing the proposal for this book, and Richard Townrow, for all his support, patience, and guidance.

# Contents

# About the author

Jane Padmore is the Deputy Director of Nursing and Quality at Hertfordshire Partnership University NHS Foundation Trust. Previously she worked in a variety of roles in CAMHS, including lead clinician, safeguarding nurse and consultant nurse in community Tiers 2 and 3, in-patient services and adolescent forensic services, as well as in multi-agency teams for looked-after children and youth offending services.

Jane has two children and two step-children, she is a back-up foster carer, and has served in various roles on the governing body, including chair, of a primary school. Her doctoral study investigated the mental health needs of young people involved in street gangs. Jane is an alumni of the Florence Nightingale Foundation, having been awarded a Travel Scholarship to enable her to explore how to translate her research into practice.

# Preface

When professionals from partner agencies and students come into contact with child and adolescent mental health services (CAMHS) and children and adolescents with mental health problems, they can find it somewhat bewildering. Decisions and actions that are taken can appear to be beyond explanation. This book is written with two primary audiences in mind. First, pre- and post-registration health and social care professionals who may be new to the field of CAMHS. The second audience is partner agencies, such as education, social care, and the voluntary sector. CAMHS is often viewed as an impenetrable 'Ivory Tower' where the decisions made are difficult to understand. This book aims to provide a broad overview that will aid understanding and give insight into the world of CAMHS.

Although mental health training is moving towards a lifespan approach to difficulties, books and training still tend to focus on adult mental health, with only a brief mention of child and adolescent mental health. Professionals of all mental health and social care disciplines may have the opportunity of a placement in CAMHS as part of their training. Arriving at a placement with a limited knowledge of how the service is configured, what it does, and what and how it assesses and treats children and young people can be overwhelming. Also, precious learning time can be taken up gaining this understanding.

Professionals in partner agencies, such as education and social care agencies, as well as the voluntary sector, frequently refer to CAMHS and often feel frustrated when referrals are not accepted or their expectations of CAMHS treatment are not met. This book seeks to clarify the language used in CAMHS as well as what can be expected from a CAMHS referral, assessment and treatment, and what legislation and policy guide the work.

The first few chapters of the book set out the contexts within which the young person lives, develops, and is involved with CAMHS. This includes a history of CAMHS, the agency and service contexts, and the context for the child, young person, and family. The book goes on to address the comprehensive CAMHS assessment and the complex areas of risk assessment and management. Finally, an overview is provided of the interventions used before conclusions are drawn and areas for future development are suggested.

# List of abbreviations

| | |
|---|---|
| ADHD | attention deficit hyperactivity disorder |
| AMHS | adult mental health services |
| ASD | autism spectrum disorder |
| CAF | Common Assessment Framework |
| CAMHS | child and adolescent mental health services |
| CAPA | Choice and Partnership Approach |
| CBT | cognitive behavioural therapy |
| CORC | Child Outcomes Research Consortium |
| CQC | Care Quality Commission |
| CRG | Clinical Reference Group |
| CYP-IAPT | Children and Young People's Improving Access to Psychological Therapies |
| DASH-13 | Desistence for Adolescents who Sexually Harm |
| DAWBA | Development and Well-Being Assessment |
| DBT | dialectical behaviour therapy |
| DOLS | Deprivation of Liberty Safeguards |
| DSH | deliberate self-harm |
| DSM V | Diagnostic and Statistical Manual of Mental Disorders V |
| EDS | eating disorder services |
| ERASOR | Estimate of Risk of Adolescent Sexual Offence Recidivism |
| ERIC | Education and Resources for Improving Childhood Continence |
| FGM | female genital mutilation |
| FPM | Family Partnership Model |
| GP | general practitioner |
| HEI | higher education institution |
| IAPT | Improving Access to Psychological Therapies |
| ICD-10 | International Classification of Diseases, tenth revision |
| IPT | interpersonal therapy |
| IPT-A | interpersonal therapy for adolescents |
| LAC | looked-after children |
| LGBT | lesbian, gay, bisexual or transsexual |
| MAOA | monoamine oxidase A |
| MAPPA | multi-agency public protection arrangements |
| MASH | Multi-Agency Safeguarding Hub |
| MFT | multiple family therapy |
| MRI | magnetic resonance imaging |
| MUPS | medically unexplained physical symptoms |

| NEET | not in education, employment or training |
| NHS | National Health Service |
| NICE | National Institute for Health and Care Excellence |
| OCD | obsessive-compulsive disorder |
| ODD | oppositional defiant disorder |
| PDD | pervasive development disorder |
| PSHE | personal, social and health education |
| PTSD | post-traumatic stress disorder |
| QNCC | Quality Network for Community CAMHS |
| QNIC | Quality Network for Inpatient CAMHS |
| SAVRY | Structured Assessment of Violence Risk in Youth |
| SDQ | Strengths and Difficulties Questionnaire |
| SEAL | Social and Emotional Aspects of Learning programme |
| SIFA | Screening Interview for Adolescents |
| SQIFA | Screening Questionnaire Interview for Adolescents |
| SSRI | selective serotonin reuptake inhibitor |
| TaMHS | Targeted Mental Health in Schools project |
| TDA | Trust Development Authority |
| YOS | youth offending service |
| YOT | youth offending team |
| YRO | Youth Rehabilitation Order |

# 1 Introduction

The aim of this book is to provide an understanding of ways of working with children and young people with mental health problems and the services available to them, and how these work. To begin to understand child and adolescent mental health problems, however, it is necessary to have some knowledge of 'normal' child development and what mental health and well-being actually mean for a child. Many theories have been developed to explain children's development and their mental health needs. This chapter provides a brief overview of child development theory and the reasons why difficulties might occur, as well as the factors that contribute to a child's resilience. A detailed account of the complex area of child development and developmental milestones is not possible here but can be found in the suggested further reading at the end of the chapter.

## Child development

The foundation for life, including mental health, is built early in life, cognitively, biologically, emotionally, sexually, and socially. The process of growth and change through life is called 'development'. Child development is an important consideration for child and adolescent mental health services (CAMHS). Disruptions or delays in achieving the milestones can be a sign that something is wrong.

Everyone experiences challenges as they walk through life and most face these without experiencing mental health problems. But there are some young people who find it hard to make the transition through childhood into adulthood, and traumatic events can trigger problems for children and young people who are already vulnerable.

Each of the main areas of development will now be looked at in turn, though it is important to understand that these should be seen not in isolation but as interacting and overlapping with one another.

### Cognitive development

As a child's cognitive development evolves, they are able to construct thought processes that include remembering, problem-solving, and decision-making. A child's cognitive development has an impact on their ability to communicate, their emotions and their behaviours, as well as their ability to engage in moral reasoning. Jean Piaget was probably the most influential voice of developmental psychology in the twentieth century.

### Biological and physical development

The brain (neuropsychiatry/psychology) and genetics are increasingly being reported as having an important part to play in a child's development. There is still much to explore and discover, particularly in relation to the result of the interaction between a child's genetic predispositions and their exposure to significant adversity in the environment. It is important to note that genes do not form a child's destiny. The genes contain instructions that tell the body how to work. The environment and the genes interact and impact how the development of the child goes forward.

Most brain development takes place in childhood and this occurs unevenly, with different parts of the brain developing at different times. This development includes visual and auditory development, language development, physical and motor development, and emotional and social development. Early experiences shape the developing brain and prolonged and severe stress can damage its architecture.

Many changes occur biologically during the journey from being a baby who is completely dependent on adults through childhood and adolescence into adulthood. With this development comes mastery of specific skills, including physical skills. As they develop, children feel the need and desire to become more independent and perform an increasing number of tasks for themselves. Each individual develops at their own rate, the reasons for which are many and varied but include the young person's experience of trauma and their cognitive ability.

### Emotional development

The emotional and mental health of children is just as important as their physical health. It assists children to develop the resilience they need to cope with whatever they will encounter in life and helps them to grow into healthy adults. Attachment theory, which is often used to explore this area of development, introduces the concept of the internal working model (Bowlby, 1969). This model explains how a child makes mental representations to understand the world, self, and others. Interaction with others and the understanding of these are guided by the memories and expectations that a child has. Through these the child's view of the world is created.

### Sexual development

Sexual development can refer to the physical changes that a child experiences as they grow up but can equally refer to their psychosexual development.

The emotional and psychological aspects of sexuality are as important as the physical changes that occur. A child will learn, explore, and experience sensation in their body; they will explore what their gender means to them and what they find attractive. They may ask endless questions and talk about having boyfriends or girlfriends.

Puberty can be a particularly challenging time for some children, as it is accompanied by a new set of experiences, questions, and hormones. Cultural and social norms and differences are all part of the personal exploration of young people.

### Social development

Social development can be understood through behaviourism and social learning theory. Erikson's psychosocial theory of child development is often used to explore this area of study. Responsive relationships with consistent primary caregivers help build positive attachments that support healthy social-emotional development. These relationships form the foundation of mental health and well-being. Disruptions in this developmental process can impair a child's capacities for learning and relating to others, with lifelong implications.

The family and parenting styles have an impact on children's development. These offer the child opportunities to socialize, test out boundaries, and learn appropriate behaviours and moral codes. These are coupled with the development of friendships, which form an important part of the social development of a child. Friendships offer companionship, security, fun, and validation. They also contribute to the child developing moral reasoning, resilience, and the ability to negotiate and resolve conflict. Young people will learn how to interact with and negotiate with people who are in positions of authority as well as with those who may be more vulnerable than them.

## Mental and emotional well-being in children and young people

There is more to good mental health than avoiding or treating mental illness. Children and young people need to be emotionally healthy and resilient and positive mental well-being is an important consideration. Also important are feelings of contentment, enjoyment, confidence, and engagement with the world, as well as high self-esteem and self-confidence. As with adults, there is a strong connection between physical, emotional, and mental well-being among the young.

Sound mental health provides a foundation for all other aspects of human development. Understanding what a mentally and emotionally healthy child looks like can assist the CAMHS clinician when working with young people. It will aid the identification of strengths and difficulties and inform the development of interventions that increase resilience. A child or young person with good mental health could be described as someone who is able to do the following (Mental Health Foundation, 2002):

- develop emotionally, creatively, intellectually and spiritually
- initiate, develop and sustain mutually satisfying personal relationships
- face problems, resolve them and learn from them in ways appropriate for the child's age
- develop a sense of right and wrong
- be confident and assertive
- be aware of others and empathize with them
- enjoy solitude
- play and learn.

Many things can contribute to a young person improving their well-being and resilience, things that can help keep children and young people mentally well. These are relevant to all children and young people, not just those with vulnerabilities or difficulties, and include physical health and well-being, nutrition and exercise, the family, education, leisure and social life, and a sense of self-esteem and confidence.

Physical health needs are as important as mental health needs when considering the emotional resilience of children and young people and they should not be considered as separate entities. They are two significant and interlinking aspects of a child's experience. Children and young people who present with behavioural, emotional or mental health difficulties often have their physical health needs overlooked. They may have been excluded from school frequently and so have missed immunizations and health checks. They may not have had any acute health needs requiring a visit to their GP, and so not have had their health reviewed since they started school.

All children and young people need a balanced and nutritious diet and should engage in regular exercise and physical activity. This is essential for good mental health, as is being part of a family that gets on well together most of the time and going to a school that is concerned for the welfare of all its pupils. Good emotional health is more likely to be maintained when there is a balance between a child being challenged and supported to keep learning and having the time and the freedom to play, both indoors and outdoors. It is also important for the child or young person to socialize and take part in activities for their age group, and spend time developing friendships and finding something that they enjoy.

Young people need to feel loved, trusted, understood, valued, and safe. If they have a warm, open relationship with their parents, children will usually feel able to tell them if they are troubled. A parent or significant adult who is able to listen and take their feelings seriously contributes to the resilience a child will develop. Children and young people can be supported to develop an interest in life and other people, recognizing what they are good at and accepting who they are. Optimism and hopefulness, as well as being able to learn from all experiences, help to increase resilience.

Although the strategic context is important to understand, it is not the only context. Chapters 2 and 3 will explore the agency and service contexts within which CAMHS teams sit, particularly in relation to historical development, social policy, and partner agencies. This is complemented by Chapter 4, which addresses the context for the child, young person, and their family.

## Key messages

- Child development can be viewed through a variety of theoretic frameworks, each of which adds something to our understanding of children and young people.
- All children and young people experience challenges and difficulties, and most navigate their way through these without experiencing mental health problems.
- Children and young people who develop emotional resilience are well equipped and are better protected against mental health problems throughout their life.

## Further reading

Berk, L. (2012) *Child Development*, 9th edn. London: Pearson.

Dwivedi, K.N. (2004) *Promoting the Emotional Well-Being of Children and Adolescents and Preventing Their Mental Ill Health: A Handbook*. London: Jessica Kingsley.

Pearce, C. (2011) *A Short Introduction to Promoting Resilience in Children* (JKP Short Introductions). London: Jessica Kingsley.

# Agency context

2

This chapter provides a general overview of CAMHS. All agencies that work with children and young people have a unique history and culture. In order to gain insight into the decisions made by and the work of CAMHS, its place strategically and among its partner agencies will be explored. This will cover the historical, legislative, political, and policy development of CAMHS.

## History

| 1920s | The 1920s saw the emergence of child psychoanalysis and child guidance. |
|---|---|
| 1989 | The United Nations Convention on the Rights of the Child (UN General Assembly, 1989) increased the awareness of the needs and rights of children, independently of those of adults.<br>    The Children Act 1989 requires that any intervention into a child's or family's life should result in the situation being demonstrably better for the child than not intervening at all. |
| Until 1990s | Child Guidance Centres overseen by the local authority. Separate inpatient services overseen by the health authority. |
| 1990s | The closure of Child Guidance Centres, and the development of community child and adolescent mental health services. The NHS oversees all child and adolescent mental health. Introduction of the four-tier model (explained in Chapter 3). |
| 1998 | The Crime and Disorder Act 1998 led to Youth Offending teams being established in each locality.<br>    Quality Protects (Department of Health, 1998) was launched with the aim of improving the life chances for looked-after children. |

| 1999 | Local Sure Start and the National Healthy Schools programmes were introduced. |
|------|------|
| 2000 | The NHS Plan Implementation Programme (Department of Health, 2000) included a requirement that health and local authorities work together to produce a local CAMHS strategy. |
| 2003 | *Every Child Matters* (DfES, 2003) was published. This came about following the inquiry into the death of Victoria Climbié (Laming, 2003). It emphasized the need for comprehensive and coordinated multi-agency working. |
| 2004 | The Children Act 2004 put the recommendations from *Every Child Matters* into statute. |
| 2009 | *New Horizons* (Department of Health, 2009) took a lifespan approach to mental health and set out a vision for improving the mental health of the whole population across the age range. |
| 2010 | Section 131A of the Mental Health Act 1983 took effect. There was a duty to provide an age-appropriate environment for young people admitted for inpatient care. |
| 2012 | *Positive for Youth* (DfE, 2012) was published to guide services for young people aged 13–19. This detailed how, where it is 'reasonably practicable', services should be offered that improve young people's physical and mental health and emotional well-being. |
| 2011 | *No Health Without Mental Health: A Cross-Government Mental Health Outcomes Strategy for People of All Ages* (Department of Health, 2011a). |
| 2013 | Commissioning of inpatient CAMHS moved from the local Clinical Commissioning Groups to NHS England. |

Discussions about emotional and behavioural problems observed by paediatricians have been conducted in the medical literature for some time. CAMHS are still in the early stages of developing the foundations for an evidence-based practice, which has led to different approaches being favoured at different times and clinicians being trained in a variety of modalities. These have included psychoanalysis, cognitive behavioural therapy, systemic therapy, mentalization, dialectic behavioural therapy and mindfulness, in addition to the use of medication, also known as psychopharmacology. All of these have their merits but developing a therapeutic relationship with the child and family is important, whatever the treatment modality.

During the late 1990s and 2000s, national policy placed increased emphasis on the idea of multi-agency and flexible working practices to help address the mental health needs of young people. Early intervention was also given increased emphasis and funding. The Children's Act 2004 provided the legal framework underpinning the recommended transformation of children's services and set out the UK Government's approach to improving the well-being of all children, providing a statutory basis to ensure services cooperate. It set out a framework for the reform of children's services.

In April 2010, significant changes were enforced for children and young people who were admitted to an inpatient service. The age-appropriate environment duty under s. 131A of the Mental Health Act 1983 took effect. This placed new responsibilities on NHS Trust Boards providing inpatient mental health services and 'places of safety' to care for children and young people separately from adults. From this time, admitting a person under 18 to an adult ward has been considered a serious incident and is reportable under the National Framework for Reporting and Learning from Serious Incidents Requiring Investigation.

The No Health Without Mental Health strategy (Department of Health, 2011a) aimed to improve the mental health of people of all ages and backgrounds and set out six objectives: (1) more people will have good mental health; (2) more people with mental health problems will recover; (3) they will have good physical health; (4) they will have a positive experience of care and support; (5) fewer people will suffer avoidable harm; (6) fewer people will experience stigma and discrimination.

## Commissioning

The commissioning of CAMHS is complex, with multiple agencies involved. The box below sets out which organization is usually responsible for commissioning which element of CAMHS.

| Commissioning body | Service |
|---|---|
| NHS England | Inpatient services<br>Services to prevent admission and facilitate discharge<br>Highly specialist outpatient services |
| Clinical Commissioning Group | Services to prevent admission and facilitate discharge<br>Tier 3 CAMHS<br>YOS health worker<br>CAMHS delivered in schools<br>Paediatric liaison |

| Local authority | Looked-after children services<br>Parenting programmes<br>Educational psychologist |
| --- | --- |
| Schools | CAMHS practitioner in the school setting<br>School counsellors<br>Educational psychologist |

Consider the impact of these complex commissioning arrangements on:

1. The CAMHS practitioner who is delivering the service.
2. The children's, young people's, and the family's experience of the services.

What risks might this pose to the care delivered?

## Quality assurance

A number of bodies are responsible for quality assurance in CAMHS, including the Commissioners, the Care Quality Commission (CQC), Monitor, the Quality Network for Inpatient CAMHS (QNIC), the Quality Network for Community CAMHS (QNCC), the Trust Development Authority (TDA), and criteria such as 'You're Welcome'.

The Commissioners have contracts with the providers of CAMHS to deliver services. Some areas have entered into joint commissioning arrangements between health, social care, and occasionally education. These contracts are monitored on an on-going basis and providers need to give assurance and evidence to the Commissioners of the quality of their service.

The Care Quality Commission, Monitor, and the Trust Development Authority all have statutory responsibilities. The Care Quality Commission is the independent regulator of health and social care in England and uses a framework for inspecting services. This framework considers whether a service is Safe, Caring, Responsive, Effective, and Well led. The Care Quality Commission also looks after the standards of care for people who are detained under the Mental Health Act. Monitor is the regulator for health services in England whose role is to make the sector work better for patients. The Trust Development Authority provides supports, oversight, and governance to all NHS Trusts to assist them to deliver what patients want. It works to ensure that services are of a high quality and are secure for the future.

The Quality Network for Inpatient CAMHS and the Quality Network for Community CAMHS are overseen by the College Centre for Quality

Improvement within the Royal College of Psychiatrists. Both provide self- and peer-reviews by members of the networks. The networks set standards with service users and these are widely used and understood. 'You're Welcome' is a framework that details the criteria that ensure that a children and young people's service is young people-friendly. This applies to all services for children and young people, not just CAMHS.

## Key messages

- CAMHS, in its current form, is a relatively young area of healthcare.
- There are complex commissioning arrangements for child and adolescent mental health services.
- Robust quality assurance frameworks are available.

## Useful websites

The Joint Commissioning Panel for Mental Health [http://www.jcpmh.info/good-services/camhs/].

'Quality Protects' Programme [http://www.york.ac.uk/res/qualityprotects/files/background.htm].

# 3 Service context

Although CAMHS can be a stand-alone service, it is usually one of many teams, professionals, and agencies working with young people and their families, each with their own language, culture, and agenda. CAMHS needs to be sensitive to this and work with partner agencies to break down barriers and build relationships. This chapter will put CAMHS into context, particularly in relation to the philosophy of care and its relationship to partner agencies.

## Philosophy of care

CAMHS is underpinned by beliefs that are based upon the nature of the child or young person and their status and rights within both the family and society. CAMHS supports the view that the child's or young person's needs should be paramount in the development of services and should provide services that are child- and young person-orientated, needs-led, research-based, adaptable, accessible, and of a high quality.

The service aims to use clinically effective interventions for children and young people experiencing mental health problems. This encompasses the assessment, diagnosis, and treatment of mental health conditions, mental health promotion, as well as training and education for service users and their families. CAMHS assists the young person and their family to prevent or manage the physiological, physical, social, emotional, and spiritual effects of a mental health problem or condition and its treatment.

CAMHS also has a strategic role in the development of local services to address the mental health needs of the local population. They also have a duty to evaluate the service they provide. This is partly done by collecting and sharing anonymized data relating to the patient group, interventions and outcomes, which is then used to evaluate the service and plan future developments.

The service has a 'duty of care' to the children and young people they see. This is the common-law obligation to exercise a level of care towards an individual, as is reasonable in all the circumstances, to avoid injury to that individual or their property. NHS organizations are liable for clinical negligence to individuals to whom they owe a duty of care. In general, NHS organizations have a duty of care to patients, service users, and visitors. The liability for a breach of that duty is based upon the relationship of the parties, the negligent act or omission, and the reasonable foreseeability of loss to that individual.

## Clinical governance

'Clinical governance is the system through which NHS organizations are accountable for continuously improving the quality of their services and safeguarding high standards of care, by creating an environment in which clinical excellence will flourish' (NHS Executive, 1999). Clinical governance is the way in which NHS organizations quality assure their services and ensure that they are safe, as well as creating the conditions for quality improvement year on year. It means creating a culture that is truly patient-centred and places quality at the top of the agenda. While clinical governance is the local manifestation of the statutory duty of quality that has been placed on all NHS organizations, it operates within a national framework for healthcare quality in which structures and mechanisms have been created and continue to evolve.

Traditionally, there have been eight pillars of clinical governance. These are patient and public involvement, patient and staff safety, clinical audit, clinical effectiveness, staffing and staff management, education, training and continuing professional development, and the use of information. More recently, these have been refined but the principles remain the same. In summary, clinical governance is everybody's business in the NHS.

## Multi-agency working

Daily, in almost every aspect of their lives, children and young people come into contact with multiple people, including professionals, who will have an impact on their mental health. The greater the concern about a young person, the more there is a tendency to increase the number of people working with that young person. This has the potential to increase the risk of conflicting measures being applied and of communication breaking down.

The Common Assessment Framework (CAF) is a generic multi-agency assessment tool for children with additional needs, which can be used by practitioners across all children's services in England. Such a framework includes a plan that is written and implemented by the Team Around the Child. The CAF aims to help early identification of need, promote coordinated service provision, and reduce the number of assessments that children go through. All local authorities were expected to implement the CAF before March 2008.

As the CAF is primarily a tool used in universal services, the implication for CAMHS can, at first, appear minimal. In practice, the CAF, and its implementation, are key to effective multi-agency working where information is shared appropriately and care is coordinated to meet the needs of children. The use of the CAF differs in each locality but CAMHS is expected to contribute to its development and be part of the Team Around the Child, often taking on the role of Lead Professional.

CAMHS needs to work closely with all other partner agencies, both statutory and voluntary, that are working with a young person and this needs to be approached with respect and a genuine desire to work together. If successful, this brings the richness of multiple perspectives and knowledge of the young person to the care and management of the difficulties. Historically, the relationship between CAMHS and other agencies has not been easy, with misunderstandings on all sides. It takes time and effort to break down the barriers and misconceptions and to develop good working relationships for the benefit of the children, young people, and their families.

The Team Around the Child, or as some areas call it the Team Around the Family, brings with it the expectation that services from all agencies will embrace the development of comprehensive, integrated, multi-agency child health services. This ought to provide seamless care across organizational boundaries, so that services can work collaboratively with families and partner agencies towards improving the outcomes for children so that they are healthy, safe, enjoying and achieving, making a positive contribution, and achieving economic well-being.

In order to work effectively across agencies, people working directly with children and young people need to have sufficient knowledge, training, and support to promote the psychological well-being of children, young people, and their families and to identify early indicators of difficulty. CAMHS and its partners often work together to develop protocols for referral, support, and early intervention that are agreed between them. Some of the partners of CAMHS are considered in the following pages.

## CAMHS partners

### Multi-Agency Safeguarding Hubs

Locally Multi-Agency Safeguarding Hubs (MASHs) have been established, which include professionals from CAMHS and adult mental health services. The principle is that referrals for additional services come through one point of contact and therefore no children can be lost by boundaries around clinical sub-teams and referral thresholds.

### Health partners

CAMHS is not the only health service that will be involved with a young person. There will also be a family doctor (GP) and health visitor (pre-school) or school nurse (of school age). Additionally, there could be speech and language therapists, paediatricians, occupational therapists, physiotherapists,

and dieticians, to name but a few. Furthermore, there are child health or paediatric practitioners and mental health practitioners with a special interest in the
mental health of children and young people with chronic medical conditions.

### Education partners

The National Institute for Health and Care Excellence (NICE) has published
two guidelines specifically on the mental health needs of young people in
schools. These are *Social and Emotional Wellbeing for Children and Young
People in Primary School* (2008a) and *Social and Emotional Wellbeing for
Children and Young People in Secondary School* (2009b). Many teachers
have difficulty identifying children who have mental health problems, so
CAMHS clinicians have been working with those in education to increase the
teachers' mental health literacy and provide services within school.

In 2005, the Social and Emotional Aspects of Learning (SEAL) programme
was introduced in primary schools. This was followed in 2007 by materi-
als for secondary schools. The Targeted Mental Health in Schools (TaMHS)
project was commissioned at a local level with teams piloting different ways
of working in schools to address the mental health needs of young people.
The final evaluation report was published in November 2011 (Department of
Health, 2011a).

### Social care partners

CAMHS and social care have a close relationship, with many of the same
young people in common. At times, there are challenges when the services
work together, often due to misunderstandings, a lack of appreciation of
each other's workload and thresholds for a service, and frequent turnover in
staff. Misunderstandings tend to occur between CAMHS and social care when
the relationship is not nurtured and supported at all levels from operational
clinicians right the way through to commissioners.

In many localities, teams have been developed that are partnerships
between the two organizations. When the services are based together in the
same building, the individual professionals can form good working relationships and develop clear protocols together. This facilitates a coordinated
approach to care that benefits the young people and their families. These
services include early intervention, youth offending services, services for
looked-after children, and services for children with disabilities.

### Youth justice partners

The aim of the youth justice system, as stipulated in the Crime and Disorder
Act 1998, is to prevent offending and re-offending by children and young
people. Youth Offending Services (YOS) are in place in every geographical

area of England and Wales. They work with 10- to 18-year-olds and include a health worker, most often a mental health worker.

As the mental health of young offenders is so relevant to the work of the YOS, it is important that YOS workers promote mental health and work towards preventing mental ill health in young people. Promoting health and detecting vulnerabilities is part of the role of all YOS staff. Dew et al. (1998) found that someone is more likely to engage professional help if another person recommends it. This would suggest that the attitudes and beliefs of YOS workers influence whether or not a young person engages with health services, not just whether they are referred to the health services in the first place.

The ASSET is a structured assessment tool that the YOS uses with every young person involved in offending behaviour, and it has a section about mental health. The young person will score highly if the mental health difficulty contributes to the offending behaviour, regardless of how severe the mental health problem is.

The Youth Justice Board for England and Wales (2011) introduced the Screening Questionnaire Interview for Adolescents (SQIFA) and, where it has been implemented, each YOS worker is responsible for completing the questionnaire with the young people allocated to them, if the young person scores significantly on the ASSET. The tool is designed to screen for mental health problems and indicates when a health referral ought to be made. The SQIFA is based on a medical model with categories separated by diagnosis (alcohol use, drug use, depression, post-traumatic stress disorder, anxiety, self-harm, attention deficit hyperactivity disorder, and psychosis).

If the SQIFA indicates that the young person requires further assessment in relation to their mental health needs, the YOS worker refers them to the YOS health worker. This worker can then complete the mental health Screening Interview for Adolescents (SIFA), which is a detailed interview. This tool is not consistently used across the youth justice system but is a useful resource for practitioners less experienced in CAMHS.

## Key messages

- The needs of the child or young person are paramount.
- Clinical governance systems ensure safe, effective, and high-quality services.
- Effective working with partner agencies, including appropriate information sharing, is essential when working with children and young people.

## Further reading

Glenny, G. and Roaf, C. (2008) *Multiprofessional Communication: Making Systems Work for Children*. Maidenhead: Open University Press.

# 4 Context for the child, young person, and family

Mental health difficulties affect approximately 10 per cent of children and young people between the ages of 5 and 16. Having a mental health problem in childhood or adolescence has been shown to increase the risk of having mental health problems as an adult. Such problems reduce the chance of success academically and socially as well as increase the risk of substance misuse, self-harm, and suicide. Early detection, intervention, and support for these children and young people are essential to protecting against this and building resilience for life. Many things can affect the mental health of a child or young person and so their whole context and environment need to be considered.

Children, young people, and their families live within their own unique context that is influenced by many, varied factors. This chapter considers these factors and how they impact on a young person's life. Clinicians need to be respectful of and sensitive to children and young people's cultural, religious, and ethnic background as well as consider their age, sexual orientation, gender, socioeconomic status, and any disability that they may have, without making assumptions based on preconceived ideas.

Socio-cultural factors, such as attitudes and beliefs, influence help-seeking behaviour and engagement in treatment. Attitudes and belief systems in a society have a major impact on the help-seeking behaviour of people suffering from mental distress via their social network. CAMHS tends to see a relatively high rate of young people who do not attend appointments. It is likely that this is due to their beliefs about mental health and the services on offer rather than their need having been resolved.

Not only does CAMHS, and its partners, reside within a context, but so too do the children, young people, and their families. There are certain risk factors that make some children and young people more vulnerable to mental health problems, such as having a long-term physical illness, parental mental illness or substance misuse, being a carer, criminogenic families, poverty, parental divorce or separation, abuse or neglect. Therefore, the context for the lives of the service users will also be considered, taking particular account of the social context.

## The young person

As with adults, young people have their own issues about CAMHS and mental health services. They may think that CAMHS is only for 'mad' people or feel ambivalent about having contact with CAMHS. They may also have significant concerns about confidentiality, particularly if they are being seen in an education setting or if they have a history of involvement with multiple agencies.

Children and young people need to trust the person they see and this does not come automatically. A therapeutic relationship needs to be established, something that is explored further in Chapter 6. The young person may have a very real concern that they may be mentally ill and be frightened of this possibility. This may lead them to ignore their condition, in the hope that it will go away. This is particularly true if they are hoping to pursue a career where a history of a mental illness might prevent them from taking up a position.

- What factors do you think increase the risk of mental health difficulties for children and young people?
- What factors do you think would increase their resilience?

## Culture and ethnicity

The importance of issues such as ethnicity, culture, and racism in relation to mental health is now well established. Fernando (1991) described how applying Western mental health paradigms across the globe may be problematic in terms of the validity, possible biases and misconceptions, and the problems and injustices that arise from clinical practice. Power, control and status, stereotyping, the young person's and their family's experience of psychiatric services, and the expression of illness, all need to be considered when working with an individual. Littlewood and Lipsedge (1997) offer a full and interesting exploration of race, culture, and psychiatry.

## Asylum seekers and refugees

Although many young refugees are extremely resilient, despite the variety of hardships they encounter, Hodes (2000) suggests that up to 40 per cent of refugee children and adolescents in the UK may be experiencing psychiatric disorders, including depression, post-traumatic stress disorder, and anxiety-related difficulties. In addition, young refugees are likely to be suffering from multiple losses and bereavements. These young people are extremely vulnerable to mental health problems due to past traumatic experiences and losses, as well as the ongoing stressors, such as uncertainty regarding their asylum application and inadequate housing. Thus, care must be taken so that normal reactions to the asylum-seeking process are not labelled as mental illness.

Unaccompanied minors are young people under the age of 18, who are outside their country of origin, separated from both parents or from their legal guardian, and applying for asylum. These young people may be referred to CAMHS and are entitled to an allocated social worker. There may be dispute about their age but CAMHS will work with the age given until proven otherwise.

These young people may not be familiar with how UK systems work, and accessing the appropriate services can be challenging due to both language and cultural differences. Translating letters is important but the service also needs to consider the young person has the ability to read and write. Interpreters may also be used because, despite the apparent ability of the young person to speak and understand English, they may feel more comfortable speaking about sensitive issues in their mother tongue and an interpreter should be provided. Another important consideration is that the terms 'mental health' and 'therapy' as they are known in Western culture may be alien concepts to a young refugee.

## English as a foreign language

Some families do not have English as their first language. Even if their English is good enough to get by in daily life, the conversations that are had in CAMHS require a person to feel comfortable and able to speak freely. A young person should never be used as an interpreter for their parents in a CAMHS appointment. CAMHS will provide and work with interpreters if they are needed. In addition, assessment reports, care plans, and letters can be translated for them. The clinician also needs to be particularly sensitive to people who may not be literate.

## Bullying

Bullying is common and unacceptable and it can seriously affect a child or young person's mental health. It can be physical or psychological and take many forms. Children and young people that present to CAMHS for assessment are often reluctant to talk about being bullied initially. They may be embarrassed or frightened of the consequences of reporting the bullying. The fear generated from bullying can result in a variety of difficulties such as school refusal, nightmares, social phobias or depression.

## The family

Families come in many varieties, can be very complex, and have their own unique culture. The CAMHS clinician needs to be mindful that what they think is 'abnormal' may in fact be perfectly acceptable in the young person's family. CAMHS clinicians gain an understanding of families through discussion and drawing a genogram with the family (genograms are explored in Chapter 7). In some families, extended family members such as grandparents or aunts or uncles might take the role of primary caregiver. And there are families who have blended through marriage, foster families, adopted families, and fractured families.

Families come with their own stories and history that may impact on the young person's mental health. The family may have genetic factors that contribute to the present situation or adverse social circumstances such as poverty, crime or illness. The young person may be aware of some of the details but the family may have decided not to keep them fully informed. This may be developmentally appropriate but the effects may still be felt by the young person.

## Looked-after children

'Looked-after children' is the term introduced by the Department of Health in 1989 to describe all children in public care, including those in foster or residential homes and those still with their parents but subject to care orders. There are two main reasons why children are looked after. They may be subject to care orders under s. 31 Children Act 1989. This means that the child has suffered or is likely to suffer significant harm without a care order. Other looked-after children are accommodated on a voluntary basis under s. 20 Children Act 1989.

Local authorities must have arrangements in place to ensure every looked-after child has their health needs assessed on entering care and has a health plan setting out how the assessed needs will be met. The health plan must be reviewed regularly. Local authorities also need to ensure that young people leaving care, as they enter adulthood, are not isolated and participate socially and economically. Young people who are or who have been looked after have higher rates of early parenthood, mental illness and stress, loneliness, and risk-taking behaviour.

About 60–70 per cent of looked-after children have a mental disorder and 20 per cent feel they have no one to talk to. There can be barriers to these children receiving CAMHS assessments and treatment. These include a lack of accurate recognition of mental health need by carers and social workers, the chaotic lifestyle the young person may lead, a lack of provision, and difficulties that come with unstable residential placements.

## Young carers

Many children and young people are carers of relatives. This may be a parent, a sibling or grandparent who has a physical or mental health condition. The needs of the child carer and the disabled or ill relative are often kept artificially separate because many services are organized to deal with individuals and not families. Children and their families are best helped when services work together and share experiences to improve outcomes. The family context needs to be considered. The impact of the hospitalization of a single, socially isolated parent has different implications from the hospitalization of a parent in a family where good quality alternative carers are on hand.

When a child or young person is a carer, they will worry and may see it as their responsibility to make their relative better. Caring for someone usually includes domestic chores, personal care, and emotional support. When the relative has a severe mental illness, the young person may be part of that person's delusional beliefs. This is of particular concern and should always be considered as a safeguarding issue.

Young carers often neglect their own needs and find it difficult to engage with services, as their caring responsibilities come first. They may be upset, isolated or ashamed of their relative's illness and may have been teased or bullied or have overheard unkind things said about them.

## Young offenders

Young offenders are aged 10–18 years and have committed a criminal offence, whether or not they have been convicted. Conduct disorders, suicide, depression, substance misuse, post-traumatic stress disorder, and attention deficit hyperactivity disorder are seen more commonly in the young offender population than in the general population.

Many young offenders are not registered with primary care and the only contact they have with health professionals is when they are in the hospital emergency department or in the criminal justice system. When young offenders appearing before a youth court were assessed, it was found 7 per cent had psychiatric problems of a nature and degree that required immediate treatment and intervention (Dolan et al., 1999). When considering detained young people, once conduct disorder had been excluded, Teplin et al. (2002) found that nearly 60 per cent of male young offenders and more than 66 per cent of female young offenders met diagnostic criteria and had diagnosis-specific impairment for one or more psychiatric disorders. This meant that the symptoms they were experiencing had an impact on their functioning.

'Young people at the interface of the criminal justice system and mental health services risk double jeopardy for social exclusion, alienation and stigmatisation' (Bailey, 1999). In addition, factors that are strongly associated with mental health problems, such as childhood trauma, in the form of abuse or loss, were more often identified in young offenders who were convicted of offences of a serious nature (Bailey, 1996).

## Information technology

Information technology is part of the lives of young people and can have both a positive and a negative impact. Access to the internet may be limited due to financial constraints or choices made by the family. Alternatively, access may be freely available but this can lead to detrimental as well as positive social interactions and experiences. The impact of technology on the lives of young people needs careful consideration and CAMHS needs to be mindful of the vast array of both helpful and unhelpful information that is available to young people. See the further reading section at the end of this chapter for internet resources offering information to (1) young people impacted negatively due to online abuse, and (2) young people and their carers about mental health difficulties.

## Conclusion

All children and young people are anxious, worried or face difficult times at some point in their lives and this is a normal part of growing up. This chapter has considered the areas that may impact on a young person's life causing anxiety or worry. With the support of family and those around the child, these difficulties often pass without any long-term effect or need for specialist involvement. Overcoming these difficulties will aid the child to become more resilient later in life.

Despite the fact that most things that happen to a child do not lead to mental health problems on their own, traumatic events can trigger problems for children and young people who are already vulnerable. Teenagers often experience emotional turmoil as their minds and bodies develop. An important part of growing up is working out and accepting who you are. Some young people find it hard to make this transition to adulthood, particularly if there are other issues for them, such as experimenting with alcohol, drugs or other substances, physical health problems, and experiencing prejudice. The next chapter will explore which services are available for children and young people when this happens.

### Key messages

- All children and young people experience difficulties and challenges as they grow up.
- Some of these difficulties and challenges increase the risk of the child or young person experiencing mental health problems.

## Further reading

Brotherton, G., Davies, H. and McGillivray, G. (2010) *Working with Children, Young People and Families*. London: Sage.

## Useful websites

Childline offers information about how to stay safe online [https://www.childline.org.uk/Explore/Bullying/Pages/social-networks.aspx].

MindEd is a free educational resource on children's and young people's mental health for all adults [https://www.minded.org.uk/].

The Royal College of Psychiatrists provides information for young people, their carers and professionals [http://www.rcpsych.ac.uk/expertadvice/youthinfo].

# 5 Child and adolescent mental health services

The cross-government strategy No Health Without Mental Health (Department of Health, 2011a) took a life span approach to mental health services but acknowledged the need to ensure children and young people are kept in mind. It stated: 'By promoting good mental health and intervening early, particularly in the crucial childhood and teenage years, we can help to prevent mental illness from developing and mitigate its effects when it does.'

This chapter provides an account of how mental health services are usually configured, although it should be noted that each locality has developed differing service configurations, particularly since promotion of the political localism agenda. It is important that children and young people are the reason services are in place, so a needs-led assessment of local services should inform developments and this should be coupled with young people being listened to, understood, and taken seriously. Effective services act as a safeguard for children and families, and a cost-effective investment over the medium to long term. Before we consider the different types of people that make up the CAMHS service and its role in child and mental health, it is worth considering the different perceptions about the service held by the child, young person, and their families.

When mental health difficulties are discussed in CAMHS, strengths are also considered because they are important in terms of resilience – but the terms 'strengths' and 'difficulties' are subjective terms. The professional or referrer may consider one area a problem or difficulty but the parents or the young person may view it as a positive aspect of their character or behaviour. There is a danger, when specifying strengths and difficulties, that they are viewed in a compartmentalized way without considering the whole picture. It would therefore be useful to keep in mind the changing nature, over time, of both strengths and difficulties.

An example of this might be a mother coming to CAMHS with her son, who was described in the referral letter as 'an aggressive boy, who it is feared may be on the periphery of criminal activity'. The referrer may have been concerned about the way the young person expressed his anger and potential risks he may pose. The CAMHS clinician could approach the assessment with the preconceived idea that this is a behavioural problem or a parenting problem. On exploration with the mother, it might be found that she thinks her son is depressed and that his perceived aggression is a strength in someone with a low mood and who lacks motivation. She might describe his aggression as assertion and him not taking any nonsense from anyone. She may also fear that her son is being labelled as an aggressive delinquent, despite not having a criminal record.

The mother may be concerned that without truly understanding her son's emotional state and his way of expressing himself, CAMHS will struggle to understand him and not be able to provide effective help. Taking the time to find out why he is being perceived as aggressive, treating his depression, and helping him to express his anger in an alternative way may be in line with the mother's aim for the intervention.

## Child and adolescent mental health is everyone's business

Child and adolescent mental health is everyone's business. Young people, friends, families, teachers, social workers, youth group leaders, GPs, and many more all play a part in promoting, preventing, identifying, and addressing a young person's mental health needs. Mental health is in not just the remit of the formal local child and adolescent mental health services. In order to achieve this, agencies need to work in partnership to maximize the chance of a positive outcome for young people.

Working together effectively to address child and adolescent mental health needs requires a reasonable level of mental health literacy. Health literacy is the 'ability to gain access to, understand and use information in ways which promote and maintain good health' (Nutbeam et al., 1993), and to maximize social, economic, and health development. There is an increased public awareness of health literacy, particularly regarding smoking, breast examination, heart disease, first aid skills, and knowing how to access health information. In comparison, mental health literacy is in its early stage of development.

Jorm et al. (1997) defined mental health literacy as 'knowledge and beliefs about mental disorders which aid their recognition, management or prevention'. Jorm (2000) describes six components to mental health literacy:

a. The ability to recognize specific disorders or different types of psychological distress.
b. Knowledge and beliefs about risk factors and causes.
c. Knowledge and beliefs about self-help interventions.
d. Knowledge and beliefs about professional help available.
e. Attitudes that facilitate recognition and appropriate help seeking.
f. Knowledge of how to seek mental health information.

Research has shown that members of the public do not recognize specific disorders or different types of psychological problems, and they differ from mental health experts in their beliefs about the causes of mental disorders and the most effective treatments (Jorm, 2000). There is widespread stigma regarding mental disorders, which causes an additional burden to those affected. These factors lead to delays in recognition and help-seeking behaviour and hinder public acceptance of evidence-based approaches to the difficulties.

With regard to children and young people, poor mental health literacy in partner agencies can lead to young people not being referred to CAMHS, as they presume young people do not want to see 'mental health' professionals. Children and young people are denied access to the evidence-based treatment that would improve their outcome. However, with the inclusion of emotional and mental health in personal, social and health education (PSHE) lessons, and the increased media attention given to raising awareness of mental health, young people frequently have better mental health literacy and a more positive view of mental health than adults.

It is important for partner agencies to increase their knowledge and skills about mental health to enable them to facilitate access to mental healthcare for the people they work with and empower them to make informed choices about their care. Failures in mental health literacy may cause problems in communication with CAMHS practitioners.

To break down professional boundaries, we need to have a shared language and understanding, as one of the barriers to working collaboratively is poor communication arising from differing professional languages and different problem perspectives. At the interface between mental health and other agencies, it is important the other agencies are clear about their expectation of CAMHS, and the role each agency will play in the care of the young person. There is a risk that unrealistic expectations may exist and ongoing communication is essential.

## CAMHS practitioners, professions, and roles

In 1994, Kurtz et al. identified problems in mental health services for children and young people, noting variations in staffing and practices. Since then, local services have put strategies in place to develop the workforce and their clinical competencies in line with evidence-based practice. The emphasis across the health service is ensuring the right people, with the right skills, are in the right place at the right time. The clinical competence of CAMHS practitioners is assured, maintained, and developed through regular clinical supervision, accessible clinical leadership at a local level, appropriate education to undertake their role in providing holistic care for children, young people and their families, and continued professional development.

Arriving at CAMHS for an assessment, a meeting or treatment can be overwhelming for young people, their families, and professionals alike. This can be exacerbated by the vast array of professional groups and job titles that are dropped into introductory conversations. In addition, psychiatrists are medical doctors and so have the title 'Doctor', but practitioners from other professionals groups will also have this title because it is an academic and clinical qualification too.

CAMHS practitioners tend to hold a professional and clinical qualification and some hold a number of different and complementary qualifications, such as a nurse who is also a cognitive behavioural therapist or a psychologist who is also a systemic therapist. Listed here are some of the more common professions and roles that are found in CAMHS but there will be local variations. Most CAMHS services will offer training placements for students from the various professional groups.

## Administrators

The administrators in CAMHS hold a key function. They will often be the first person someone contacting the service will speak to on the telephone or meet when they arrive at the clinic. There are numerous roles that they undertake, including receptionist, business manager, secretary, and personal assistant to an individual or a group of clinical staff. Administrators will often relay messages to clinicians and ensure reports and letters are sent out in a timely manner.

## Dieticians

Dieticians are not commonly found in CAMHS, apart from eating disorder services, but can be a valuable resource. The dietician will assess the young person's dietary and nutritional intake and then develop, with the multi-disciplinary team, a re-feeding and maintenance plan. CAMHS may refer young people to a dietician that is based outside the service if there is concern about weight gain, weight loss or nutrition for those without an eating disorder. This may be particularly important if a young person is prescribed medication that is known to cause weight gain.

## Nurses

Nurses are registered health practitioners whose names appear on the Nurse and Midwifery Council register. They can be registered as general health, mental health, learning disabilities or sick children nurses. Some are registered under multiple sections and so could be, for example, a mental health nurse and a sick children's nurse. Most CAMHS nurses are mental health nurses but other nurses may also work in CAMHS, particularly in neurodevelopment teams where learning disability nurses are often employed.

Nurses can have a number of job titles. The most common are as follows:

- *Consultant nurses or nurse consultants* are the most senior clinical nurses whose job is to teach and supervise others, assess and treat young people independently or as part of a multi-disciplinary team, and undertake research and other academic work.

- *Advanced nurse practitioners* are senior nurses with advanced knowledge in specific areas of practice. This might mean they are non-medical prescribers or that they assess and treat independently.
- *Clinical nurse specialists* are also senior nurses who are trained and have specialist knowledge in a particular area of practice or type of disorder, such as attention deficit hyperactivity disorder.
- *Community psychiatric nurses* are mental health nurses who work primarily in the community. This is a title normally used in adult services but it is occasionally used in CAMHS, particularly in early intervention psychosis teams.
- *Ward managers* are usually nurses who manage either one or a group of inpatient units. They are responsible for the day-to-day running of the ward and ensure that all aspects of the service come together to provide a high quality of care for the young person. The ward manager will usually manage the multi-disciplinary team and the charge nurses.
- *Charge nurses* are senior nurses on the ward who are responsible for managing a ward, coordinating admissions and discharges, and overseeing the nursing staff. They will also manage a group of nurses.
- *Staff nurses* are registered nurses who work on an inpatient unit. They are usually responsible for a group of young people during a shift. Newly qualified nurses will sometimes be called *preceptor nurses*.

### Primary mental health practitioners/workers

Primary mental health practitioners are clinicians from an array of different disciplines, who are allocated to a specific geographical area, based in community settings. They may have a GP or a group of GP practices to which they are linked. They are usually the first point of contact for any discussion or new referral, about a child, from anyone in their locality, particularly if there is not a central referral system. They have generic child and adolescent mental health skills and will assess young people, offer short-term treatment, and facilitate access to other local CAMHS.

### Psychiatrists

Psychiatrists are medically qualified and registered doctors who work in the field of mental health. They will sometimes be referred to as the 'doctor'. Child and adolescent psychiatrists have gone on from their basic medical training to specialize in working with young people with mental health problems and their families.

The most senior psychiatrists are *consultant child and adolescent psychiatrists*. Some of these are dual trained and registered because they have specialized in more than one area. For example, *consultant forensic child and adolescent psychiatrists* work with young people with mental health problems who are also involved in offending behaviour.

## Psychologists

Psychologists are trained to assess and help with a person's psychological functioning, emotional well-being, and development, the most senior of which are *consultant psychologists*. There are different types of psychologists who work with children and young people:

- *Clinical child psychologists* receive a different training from educational psychologists and forensic psychologists. They have been trained to understand and work with children and young people, using and applying scientific knowledge to deliver psychological interventions.
- *Educational psychologists*, in contrast, promote the learning of all children. They offer consultation, advice, and training on how schools and families can help children to learn effectively, and to make the most of their education.
- *Forensic psychologists* work specifically with young people (and adults) involved in the criminal justice system. They use their knowledge of the brain, emotions, and behaviour to understand why someone has committed a crime, what the future risks are, and how to prevent future offending behaviour.

## Social workers

As with other professional groups, different types of social worker are involved in CAMHS. Local authorities employ some social workers, whereas others are employed directly by the NHS. They are specialists who work closely with young people and families to support them either through crises or in the longer term.

- *CAMHS social workers* work as part of the CAMHS team and can work as a generic CAMHS practitioner in community services.
- *Hospital social workers* have a specific role in inpatient services, including liaising with social care, and act as the approved mental health practitioner when needed under the Mental Health Act. Others work in paediatric hospitals alongside the CAMHS paediatric liaison services and disability social workers. Hospital social workers help the young person with the social aspects of admission to and discharge from hospital.
- *Disability social workers* work in the community and ensure that children and young people with disabilities receive the social care support they need to manage their day-to-day life in the community.

- *Child protection social workers* help young people who are in danger of being abused or neglected. They assess situations where abuse or neglect is suspected and take the necessary action.
- *Looked-after children social workers* work closely with child protection social workers when a child or young person is voluntarily accommodated or removed from their home. They work to support the child in their placement and, where possible, aim for the child to return home. In some circumstances, the social worker acts on behalf of the local authority who is the 'corporate parent'.
- *Youth offending social workers* work with youngsters aged 10–18 years who are involved in the youth justice system, through assessment, writing pre-sentence reports, and managing court orders. They work with young people to address the underlying factors leading to and maintaining the offending behaviour. Their aim is to reduce the risk of reoffending and harm to the public. These social workers also support and manage young people while in court and as they move to and from custody.

## Support workers

Some members of CAMHS staff who work with young people and their families do not hold a professional qualification and registration. These roles have numerous names and functions and can be in the community or inpatient settings. They may be called community support workers, nursing assistants, family support workers or care assistants.

## Therapists

Therapist is a generic term used to describe someone who is trained to offer an assessment and treatment in a specific type of therapy. Some therapies have a stronger and more developed evidence base for efficacy than others but this may be because robust studies have not been carried out with the other therapies. Some CAMHS will only employ individuals trained in therapies for which there is evidence of its efficacy with child and adolescent mental health. Others will embrace a wide range of therapies based on their experience of whether it has been helpful. The term therapist may sometimes be substituted with psychotherapist, for example, art psychotherapist or systemic psychotherapist.

- *Art therapists* include art, music, and drama therapists. They are trained to use their medium of art to work with the young person and their subconscious. They will help the young person to find a way of expressing their complex and confusing emotions, which they may not feel able to express verbally.

- *Child psychoanalytic psychotherapists* are trained therapists who help children to deal with their emotional and mental health problems. They often use unstructured sessions at a regular time and place, allowing the child to express their complex feeling and emotions. The therapist offers insight into the child's subconscious world.
- *Family or systemic therapists* are trained to work with children and their families together, to help them understand and manage the difficulties facing them. They tend to work with the whole family, allowing them to express difficult feelings and thoughts safely. These therapists will help the family to see things from other people's perspectives and to build on their strengths.
- *Occupational therapists* work on the principle that occupation is essential to a young person's existence and to their good health and well-being. Occupation means all the things that people do or participate in, such as working, learning, caring, playing, and interacting. They are an essential part of the inpatient multi-disciplinary team, but also offer valuable assessments and interventions in the community.
- *Play therapists* work with a child using play. The child communicates through their play to the therapist. The therapist works with dynamic processes and the child explores at his own pace and with his own agenda.
- The evidence base for including a *speech and language therapist* in CAMHS is growing, particularly in neurodevelopmental services and with young offenders. These therapists are concerned with the management of disorders of speech, language, and communication.

**Other roles**

- Do you think that all roles are profession-specific or are some generic, where any profession can undertake them?
- Are they profession- or competency-led?

Some CAMHS have generic posts called *mental health practitioners* or *CAMHS practitioners*. These are open to any clinician who holds a professional registration and the appropriate training. They usually offer a generic service and assess and treat young people with their families or alone.

Other roles that are found in CAMHS are care coordinator, key worker, and lead professional. All these indicate that the clinician is the person who coordinates the care and ensures that the young person's needs are kept central. They are usually responsible for making sure that others involved in the care of the young person are aware of the work CAMHS is doing. When the Mental Health Act is used, there are specific roles that need to be fulfilled under the legislation. These are the *responsible clinician, approved clinician*, and *approved mental health practitioner.* An approved mental health practitioner may be a social worker, nurse, occupational therapist or psychologist who has undergone specialist training, and who has been approved by the local authority to act in the role; the post cannot be taken by a medical practitioner. The responsible clinician and approved clinician can be a doctor, nurse, occupational therapist, psychiatrist, psychologist or social worker. The approved clinician is a person approved to act as a clinician for the purposes of the Mental Health Act. The responsible clinician is the approved clinician with overall responsibility for the young person's care.

## Overview of service configurations

There are two approaches to service configuration in CAMHS: *tiers 1–4* or *universal, targeted, and specialist*. In reality, most localities combine the two in addition to the Children and Young People's Improving Access to Psychological Therapies (CYP-IAPT), which is increasingly available nationally. Despite child and adolescent mental health being everyone's business, there is a still a place for CAMHS, but what this looks like in each locality will vary enormously. This is complicated by frequent service redesigns to meet cost improvement programmes and a high turnover of staff. Each area's variation will have resulted from local historical factors, the political agenda, a needs analysis, as well as custom and practice. Traditionally, the tiered approach has been used but in some localities the universal, targeted, and specialist CAMHS model is preferred. However, it is likely that there is a mixture of the two approaches.

### Tiers 1–4

The tiered system is frequently referred to by CAMHS practitioners, but is often a confusing concept for those not working in the service. It is also complicated by the many interpretations of the meaning and role of the tiers. Some areas have workers who are in one tier and work there all week, whereas others have people who work in tier 3 but do a proportion of the week in tier 2.

- *Tier 1* refers to the professionals who undertake social, emotional, and developmental support, but are not part of specialist CAMHS. In general, it is not their primary role, but is an important part of the local child and adolescent mental health provision.
- *Tier 2* refers to specialist CAMHS workers using their individual professional skills with children and families for short-term interventions, where there is not currently the need for a multi-disciplinary team. The CAMHS practitioners in tier 2 require a level of experience and seniority so that they can work without the immediate support of other CAMHS colleagues. Tier 2 services tend to be located in schools or other community services.

- *Tier 3* services are multi-disciplinary CAMHS where teams of clinicians work together to assess and treat young people and their families. Tier 2 and 3 services offer consultation and training to tier 1 services, and local protocols are sometimes in place to assist this process.
- *Tier 4* services are either inpatient services for children and young people or highly specialist outpatient services. These outpatient services will usually offer a second opinion service and an assessment and treatment service for rare or complex difficulties. An example of this might be an eating disorder service that offers multi-family therapy for families, with professionals who have expertise in this area. These services are usually more cost-effective for local commissioners, due to the low level of demand in the local area, when centralized. In some cases, these services are centrally commissioned by NHS England (2014b).

### Universal, targeted, and specialist

This model has developed alongside, and uses the same language as, the social care model of service delivery. Universal services work with all children and young people, whereas targeted services provide early interventions for vulnerable children and young people. These vulnerable groups tend to be ones that are priorities for the local authority, such as looked-after children, young offenders, and those on a child protection plan. They are founded on the principle of integration through a high level of communication and joint working between partner agencies. Specialist services work with children and young people with complex, severe or persistent difficulties.

- When considering the two CAMHS models, which do you prefer and why?
- How would you combine the two models to ensure children, young people, and their families are getting a high-quality service that meets their needs?

## CAMHS teams

CAMHS is configured in many different ways across the UK. Some localities have just one team while others have multiple teams. Some localities have opted to have one main service divided into sub-teams. These may consist of a small number of clinicians working generically for the majority of the week but spending one or two days in a more specific and specialized field the rest of the time. We will now consider some of the types of teams found in CAMHS in different regions of the UK.

### Children and Young People's Improving Access to Psychological Therapies programme

Improving Access to Psychological Therapies (IAPT) is an NHS programme offering interventions, approved by the National Institute of Health and Clinical Excellence (NICE), for treating people with depression and anxiety disorders. The government gave a commitment to expand IAPT to children and young people in their *Talking Therapies: A Four-Year Plan of Action* (Department of Health, 2011b).

The Children and Young People's Improving Access to Psychological Therapies programme (CYP-IAPT) was launched in 2011. Unlike adult services, CYP-IAPT does not create stand-alone services; instead, it brings together partner agencies from a local area. These CAMHS Partnerships become part of a Learning Collaborative and include a higher education institution (HEI). The HEI provides training to existing CAMHS staff by following the CYP-IAPT national curriculum. This curriculum is not mandated; instead, it is developed locally in order to meet the needs of the local community.

Routine outcome monitoring is undertaken session by session with the aim of improving the quality and experience of services. This data has to have a direct meaning in the clinical encounter and be able to assist in the analysis of the outcomes of the service.

A critical element of CYP-IAPT is the participation of the children, young people, and their families. Systems have been put in place to enable them to contribute to the design, delivery, and monitoring of the service. Action is taken as a result of this contribution to improve the service and good practice is shared.

### CAMHS in education settings

In some areas, CAMHS services delivered directly in the education setting have been developed. These may be commissioned directly by a school or cluster of schools; others may be part of a locality-wide provision or a pilot project. The CAMHS clinician in these services usually works alone, but has a 'home' CAMHS team they are in regular contact with for support and joint working arrangements.

In schools, these clinicians are able to provide drop-in clinics for pupils and consultation clinics for staff. They can offer help with specific issues relating to individual pupils and their families, such as short-term treatment packages and group programmes. They attend annual reviews for children on school action and school action plus, and joint meetings between parents and teachers. They can facilitate referrals and access to specialist CAMHS, and network with other services and practitioners involved in working with children and young people to create more integrated services. These clinicians may also be asked to provide evidence when a statement of educational needs is being applied for.

On a more generic level, the CAMHS practitioner can provide input into the personal, social, and health education (PSHE) curriculum, deliver mental health promotion, generally promote emotional and behavioural well-being and, where possible, prevent difficulties arising. They also provide training and support to teachers. This may be formal training as an inset day or informal discussion as the need arises.

### Looked-after children CAMHS

As the name implies, CAMHS looked-after children (LAC) services offer a service to children who are 'looked after'. Each service is commissioned locally and so the population they serve may be slightly different. The team works closely with social care, foster carers, and children's homes, offering assessment, treatment, and consultation. Some LAC CAMHS offer training and support to foster carers, including formal programmes such as Treatment Foster Care and the Fostering Changes Programme. These are evidence-based interventions aimed at improving the confidence of the foster carer and promoting placement stability.

### CAMHS and youth offending services

Many young people who offend have presented with problems to a range of authorities over a period of time. Historically, the uncoordinated approaches to working with children and young people meant that services were not always made available to them prior to their offending behaviour escalating in frequency and severity.

In order to prevent offending, a holistic picture of the young person must include their mental health needs. Youth offending teams (YOTs) or youth offending services (YOS), as they are now known, were formed following the implementation of the Crime and Disorder Act 1998. These are multi-agency teams that include health, social care, probation, police, education, housing, and substance misuse services, as well as youth workers. Each agency aims to work together towards the same goal and brings a unique perspective and quality in relation to how to achieve this aim.

The youth justice system intervenes in the lives of young people to prevent offending behaviour escalating, and the Youth Justice Board requires that all YOT clients have unhindered access to health assessments. The YOS health worker's role therefore is to ensure that both the physical and mental health needs of young offenders are addressed.

Usually, the CAMHS practitioner in the YOS will be based on the site with the rest of the YOS multi-agency team, but will have strong links back to the local CAMHS. The CAMHS practitioner will offer consultation to the YOS workers and deliver training as well as assess young people and facilitate their access to local services. Some offer short-term treatment in the YOS environment, but caution is needed because young people can feel coerced into seeing a health worker, as the rest of the appointments there are mandatory. The issues of consent, capacity, and confidentiality are as applicable within the YOS setting as they are within local CAMHS.

The level of mental health needs within the young offender population is higher than in the general population. These difficulties may cause, contribute to or be a result of their offending behaviour. The YOS can work together with healthcare professionals to maximize engagement in treatment.

## CAMHS paediatric liaison teams

Children and young people with chronic, long-term physical health problems are more likely to experience mental health difficulties. These mental health problems can lead to poor compliance with treatment plans, and feelings of despair and low mood in the young person. It can also lead to behavioural difficulties and an increase in self-harm and suicide attempts. In order to address this, some paediatric services have CAMHS paediatric liaison integrated into their services.

In some areas, these CAMHS paediatric liaison services also provide emergency input into the accident and emergency department. By doing this young people who present as having self-harmed, or where there are concerns about their mental health needs, can be seen quickly. In many areas, an on-call service is provided to the department 24 hours a day, seven days a week.

## CAMHS in primary care

Some primary care practices will commission a service from the local CAMHS. This usually means that the patients from the practice will not have to wait to be seen by tier 3 CAMHS, and can be seen in the local surgery. The CAMHS practitioner will usually have links with the local CAMHS team and so be able to facilitate access to a multi-disciplinary team if needed. This CAMHS clinician will offer assessment and time-limited treatment interventions.

## Generic 0–18 CAMHS

Most localities will have a generic CAMHS for 0–18-year-olds, although some areas have not yet been able to establish a service for 16- and 17-year-olds, despite clear directives indicating that this should be the case. In these areas, there can be difficulties in identifying who is providing services for the 16–17-year-olds, resulting in this group of young people not receiving the service they require.

Generic services for 0–18-year-olds will have developed referral criteria and protocols that partner agencies can request. These will have been negotiated with the commissioners of the service and be responsive to the local needs assessment. These CAMHS teams will work closely with the other CAMHS in the locality and it is not unusual for some clinicians to work part-time in this team and part-time in another, such as the YOS or the team for looked-after children.

Some localities divide the service into smaller teams that focus on specific age groups. These teams include early years CAMHS teams who work with children who are pre-school age, children's CAMHS who work with primary school-aged children, and adolescent teams who work with secondary school-aged children. Special local arrangements are put in place if siblings fall into two or more teams. If services have this configuration, robust protocols will need to have been put in place because as children get older they cross into the age group of another team. In most cases, unless there is a long-term treatment need, the young person will finish their treatment where they started it.

## Neurodevelopment teams

Neurodevelopment teams see children with difficulties relating to their brain development. This usually involves children and young people with social communication difficulties, in combination with aspects of their behaviour that are repetitive or stereotyped and which are causing impairment. They may also see children and young people with poor attention, who are over-active and impulsive, which are noticeable in more than one setting, and are causing at least moderate impairment.

Prior to the age of 5, developmental paediatricians will usually take the lead for children who have been referred for a primary developmental problem such as speech and language delay or a suspected learning disability. When assessments take place in CAMHS neurodevelopmental teams, a medical examination and testing are usually included, and local protocols will have been developed with developmental paediatricians. This may involve an electroencephalogram, magnetic resonance imaging, checking head circumference, and chromosomes, including fragile X syndrome.

Intervention will not cure the difficulties, but will assist the young person and their family to have the information and support they need, and to manage any difficulties that may arise. This may involve seeing the family alone or with other families, and include advice on the implication of the diagnosis and appropriate management strategies and how to minimize the impact of the neurodevelopmental problems. Evidence-based treatment will be provided that will address co-morbid mental and medical disorders.

## Eating disorder services

Eating disorder services (EDS) usually cover a larger geographical area than the local CAMHS, and see only young people with anorexia nervosa and bulimia nervosa. Very few EDS will see young people with difficulties relating to obesity. The EDS offer specialist treatment for eating disorders that includes attending to their physical health as well as their mental health needs. Treatments are delivered through the young person's own family members working together to improve the situation, or multiple families working together.

### Forensic CAMHS teams

Forensic CAMHS teams, other than those in the YOS, are stand-alone services that tend to serve a regional area. Local services will frequently refer to these teams for a consultation or a second opinion with regard to an assessment and the management of risk. These teams will also provide assessment and treatment recommendation reports, fitness to plea reports for court purposes, and opinions for court.

### Early intervention in psychosis

Early intervention in psychosis services are usually adult mental health services, but are important to CAMHS as they can assess and treat young people as young as 14. The professionals in these teams are not generally trained or experienced with adolescents, so local arrangements are sometimes put in place to co-work and offer consultation. Some areas will have a CAMHS practitioner placed one or two days a week in the team.

### CAMHS early intervention

Models of early intervention vary from one locality to another. They tend to offer brief treatment to children and young people who have mental health difficulties, aimed at preventing the difficulties becoming more severe and long term. This generally means that there is a single defined mental health problem that can be treated by one mental health professional in conjunction with other agencies, rather than a multi-disciplinary health team. This would be suitable when, following assessment, it is thought that the level of risk to the child, family, and general public from their mental health problem is low to medium and a brief intervention would likely be helpful.

Prevention and early intervention delivered to children and adolescents can reduce the burden on adult services. It could be argued that if there is early intervention with adolescents, it would be cost-effective in the long term.

## Inpatient and residential child and adolescent services

A minority of children and young people spend some time as a resident in an institution. This can be as a patient in a child and adolescent mental health unit, as a prisoner within the youth justice system, as a resident in a children's home or as a pupil at a boarding school. Being a pupil at a boarding school usually means the young person has access to a school nurse and a GP, so will not be discussed here. The other three services might see mental health as a core purpose of their service whereas others may have a dedicated CAMHS within the institution.

## Child and adolescent mental health inpatient services

Inpatient services for children and adolescents have developed over time in a way that means the type of service delivered and the care pathways followed vary across the country. The majority of inpatient units are for adolescents, most of which are for those over 14 years of age. There are only a few units for primary school-age children.

Some inpatient services have specific remits, such as low secure inpatient units, adolescent psychiatric intensive care units, eating disorder wards, inpatient learning disability services, children's units, and autistic spectrum disorder services. The secure forensic mental health services are planned and commissioned through a national network. Services for the deaf are also nationally commissioned, and are covered by the Clinical Reference Group (CRG).

Recently, there have been concerns about the capacity of the services nationally in relation to demand, the distance young people and their families have to travel, and the inequality that is apparent across the country. Most child and adolescent mental health inpatient services are commissioned centrally and so, in July 2014, NHS England (2014b) published a review of the service that is provided nationally. The challenges for young people when they are not accommodated close to home can mean that visits from family are fewer and contact with social networks are reduced. The usual practice of gradual discharge, with home and school visits, is not possible and involvement of tier 3 in the care leading to discharge is reduced.

### Referrals and admission

Children and young people should only be admitted to hospital when it is the best therapeutic option for them, which usually means that there is appropriate and safe option in the community. This may occasionally be against the wishes of their parents or may be under a section of the Mental Health Act, which is considered in Chapter 7. Some localities offer an assertive outreach service to young people when the tier 3 CAMHS is considering an inpatient admission. The aim of the service is to provide intensive treatment in the community to prevent admission.

Practice varies in relation to how and what needs to take place before a young person is admitted to a ward. Admissions can be planned or unplanned but most units will require that the young person is assessed by tier 3 CAMHS, as a minimum. The only exception to this is if they present at the emergency department and are admitted from there. Some will insist that a psychiatrist is involved in the assessment, and a few will insist it is a consultant psychiatrist. When it is not an emergency, the pre-admission assessment is carried out in some areas by the tier 4 service themselves, who will visit the young person.

All inpatient services will have a documented admission protocol that stipulates their referral criteria. They will also provide information leaflets about the service designed to meet the developmental needs of the young people the unit serves. In addition, there will be information leaflets for the parents.

Young people are generally admitted to an inpatient unit because the risks they present, *due to their mental health problem*, are too high to be managed in the community. Alternatively, they may require intensive treatment or a period of time where they are observed 24 hours a day to aid the assessment.

### Ward environment

Units may be mixed sex, but the sleeping areas must be separated along the lines of gender. The sleeping arrangements for young people who are transgendered are based on a discussion with the young person and local protocols.

When a young person is being considered for admission, consideration is given to the mix of patients on the unit and their difficulties. At times negotiations will take place between units so that risks can be managed effectively. The ward environment is an important consideration for inpatient CAMHS services. Children's wards for primary school-aged children and adolescent wards for secondary school-aged children need to be developmentally appropriate. These young people are very vulnerable and away from home, in an alien environment, with other young people who are distressed, talking to people they do not know, and isolated from their social networks.

### Treatment

The assessment and treatment of children and young people on inpatient wards are regularly reviewed by a multi-disciplinary team to ensure treatment is provided that is responsive to the changing needs of the young person and their family. This team is based on the unit so that multiple perspectives can be considered and multi-faceted treatment plans delivered.

Most inpatient settings have a day programme that is adapted according to the needs of the current patients. Not every young person will be well enough to engage in this fully from the outset. Monday to Friday involve attendance at the school hospital, which may be attached to the unit, and therapy programmes. At weekends, activities are also arranged, but usually young people will spend increasing periods of time at home as they head towards discharge. Also, young people may travel to their home or school, for short periods, as they move towards discharge. The school hospital provides a valuable service in supporting this process, ensuring that the home or school understands the young person's needs and vulnerabilities.

Treatment programmes are delivered both on a one-to-one basis and in groups. They follow the best evidence base available and are aimed at recovery and relapse prevention. Risk management plans are put in place for the young person and other people's safety on the unit, but also for when they are on leave from the unit or discharged. Treatment plans involve a multidisciplinary approach and include medication management, social and life skills training, educational reintegration and family work, and on-going support in addition to care pathway specific treatments.

### Discharge

Discharge from an inpatient setting can be challenging. A lack of resources in tier 3 CAMHS can mean that the support needed to prevent a readmission is lacking. Also, although a young person may be ready for discharge in relation to their mental health problems, other circumstances may result in significant delays, such as the family's inability to cope, housing problems or lack of education provision. These delays to discharge can have a negative impact on the young person leading to them becoming institutionalized.

Supported discharge services for young people have been developed in some localities. These are services for young people who are currently inpatients. The aim is to facilitate and support young people and their families to have an earlier discharge than would normally be the case. The clinicians in this team can provide more intensive treatment, with more frequent visits than the usual community team.

### Other institutions

Young offenders institutions, secure training centres, and secure children's homes are institutions where children are living away from home, in secure settings, most often against their wishes and desires. Children and young people in these environments are significantly more likely to experience mental health problems. In response to this, services have been developed, either in-house or visiting, that provide CAMHS to these children.

It is essential that the services involved in the secure setting liaise closely with the community team. Young people who are released from these settings are often extremely vulnerable, and will be at high risk of disengaging from services on release.

## Key messages

- Child and adolescent mental health is everyone's business.
- There is a need to promote good mental health early to minimize the risk and effects in later life.

- Local services have developed in response to local needs and commissioning arrangements.
- CAMHS practitioners come from many different professional groups.

## Further reading

Bazyk, S. (ed.) (2011) *Mental Health Promotion, Prevention, and Intervention with Children and Youth: A Guiding Framework for Occupational Therapy.* Bethesda, MD: AOTA Press.

Williams, R. and Keerfoot, M. (2005) *Child and Adolescent Mental Health Services: Strategy, Planning, Delivery, and Evaluation.* Oxford: Oxford University Press.

# 6 CAMHS processes

This chapter provides an overview of the structures that guide and support the work within CAMHS, areas that can sometimes cause frustration for partner agencies. The first step a young person takes into CAMHS is usually via a referral, either by another professional or a self-referral. This is followed by a request for more information or an assessment, if the referral is accepted as being appropriate.

To make the best assessment of the young person's needs, a therapeutic relationship with the young person and their family needs to be developed. The referral, therapeutic relationship, and questionnaires are each explored in turn. This is followed by an exploration of consent and capacity, two areas that guide how clinicians work with the young people and their families. Finally, confidentiality, information-sharing, and general communication are considered in relation to the young person, their family, and partner agencies with CAMHS.

## Referral

Sometimes, making a referral to CAMHS can be a challenge. Stereotyping, perceptions of what mental health services do, and concerns about 'medicalizing' distress can lead to resistance on both the part of the referrer and the young person and their family. In addition to these challenges, each CAMHS will show subtle differences in what they are commissioned to provide, referral pathways, and available information about the service. It is the job of local CAMHS to ensure that information about inclusion and exclusion criteria and referral pathways is accurate and accessible, but this process can be improved if partner agencies work with local CAMHS to form good working relationships and protocols, as well as informal networks.

CAMHS assessments usually begin with the referral, either by another professional or a self-referral – that is, by the young person and their family. Not all CAMHS accept self-referrals, due to how they have been commissioned or local agreements. Local CAMHS are usually made up of a number of small teams, sometimes in one base but more frequently spread across a locality. This makes it a challenge to know which team to refer to, and leads to referrals being passed around teams, causing delays.

Nationally there is now a move towards a single point of access in each locality, with details about how to refer held on both NHS and local authority websites. In some localities, these are CAMHS-only referral points but in other areas there is a single point of access for all services for children. This can be a barrier to care if a young person wants to be seen by CAMHS without other agencies knowing that a referral has taken place, and so a protocol for this situation is normally developed alongside a multi-agency single access point.

The acceptable methods of referral can differ from area to area, with some only accepting one form, whereas others are more flexible. These methods include a standardized referral form devised by CAMHS, a Common Assessment Framework form, online forms, letters, telephone calls, emails, electronic forms, and walk-ins. Whatever the method, unless urgent, most services require a documented referral.

The quality and type of information contained in the referral will assist the CAMHS practitioners when they decide whether the referral meets the criteria for the service, and how urgent the need is to see the young person. Consent from the young person or the person with parental responsibility has to have been given for the referral to be made, and should be clearly documented in the referral letter. CAMHS will want to be clear who holds parental responsibility, and this should also be clearly stated. Consent is explored later in this chapter.

Referrals often state that the difficulties that a young person is experiencing are urgent in nature, for example, potential exclusion from school. This is understandably considered a priority and matter of urgency by the school and family. For CAMHS, this may raise the priority of the case, but it is unlikely that the young person will be seen urgently. Urgency in CAMHS is usually determined by an acute mental disorder, such as psychosis, or the risk that the young person poses to self or others, such as deliberate self-harm, very low body weight, or violence due to a possible mental health problem.

If the referrer provides clear and full information, CAMHS is able to make a more accurate decision about how urgently to treat the referral, who the most appropriate clinician is, and whether more information is needed. It could be argued that without the appropriate information, the referral could be rejected, when it is actually a wholly appropriate referral, leading to significant delays in the young person receiving assessment and the treatment they need.

The referral needs to state clearly what the referrer is expecting from the referral, what the reason for the referral is, and what the mental health concerns are. Issues relating to risk need to be detailed clearly alongside any plans that have been put in place to manage that risk in the interim. The referrer and the family may have tried a number of interventions or assessments already, or there may already be some form of therapy in place; this is useful information and relevant reports can be copied into the referral letter. If the person is already receiving therapeutic input, CAMHS will want to liaise with the therapist to ensure that the work currently being done is not undermined. Consent will need to be obtained to do this.

Essential information includes the risk of harm to self and others. Other information that is helpful includes any recent changes or significant issues relating to the young person's emotional state, substance use, physical health, social circumstances or behaviour, as well as any mental health or substance misuse problems in the family.

In CAMHS, referrals are received on a daily basis, and there is usually a duty system in place. Upon presentation, a clinician screens referrals and determines whether any immediate action is required. Each CAMHS will have a protocol about how they manage referrals. These protocols usually include the duty CAMHS practitioner reading the referral and taking appropriate action. They are sometimes offered support by a duty senior clinician and duty manager.

Either the whole team or a selection of clinicians and a manager attend referral meetings. It can be helpful for partner agencies to know at what time and on what day the referral meeting takes place, so that they can coordinate when they send referrals. The time prior to the referrals meeting can be used to gather information and liaise with professionals and the family to ensure that enough information is gathered to make the appropriate decision.

Decisions at the referrals meeting are documented in the clinical records, and the referrer and family are sent a letter detailing the outcome of the referrals meeting. The recipients of these letters can expect to be told how long the wait for the assessment is expected to be and what to do in the meantime if matters deteriorate or they have any questions. Alternatively, in more urgent situations, the letter will advise of an appointment time.

Referrals to inpatient services are via the community services or an emergency referral from the emergency department of an acute hospital. They rarely come directly from the general practitioner or as self-referrals, and inpatient teams would usually ask for community services to make an initial assessment in order to determine if an alternative to inpatient care is a viable option. The process for admission to inpatient services was explored in the previous chapter.

## The therapeutic relationship

The foundation – and arguably the most important part – of any effective and helpful piece of work in CAMHS is the therapeutic relationship. Young people and their families are referred to CAMHS because the professionals who comprise the service are seen as experts in child and adolescent mental health.

There is often a misconception that there are clear answers to each and every mental health problem, and a feeling that CAMHS has a magic wand to solve all the emotional ills of the world. In reality, CAMHS are working with the best available evidence at that point in time. There are many unanswered questions, new evidence is continuously being presented, and practice is evolving. Each young person and their family are unique and no one size fits all. CAMHS practitioners bring their experience in the field and knowledge of the current evidence base to the relationship, but the young person and their family are the experts in their culture, their experiences, and what has helped or not helped in the past.

The therapeutic relationship has to be developed, which is done through respect, partnership, and both verbal and non-verbal communication skills that are closely related and interlinked. Non-verbal communication can give validity to the verbal communication or, equally, can disqualify it. A thorough and evidence-based model that is used for developing and working with a therapeutic relationship is the Family Partnership Model (FPM; Davis and Day, 2010; Day et al., 2015). The FPM enables practitioners to develop effective partnerships with parents and use a structured and flexible relational, goal-orientated approach to achieve the best possible outcome while using the disorder-specific evidence base that is available.

### The expert versus the partnership model

At present, the emphasis in health is on evidence-based practice, which is aided by organizations such as the National Institute for Health and Care Excellence (NICE) and the Cochrane Database. There is an assumption that meta-analyses of controlled trials and the dissemination of clinical practice guidelines are sufficient to improve clinical practice, but this approach alone fails to take into account the views of the public in general, including those of young people and their families. If the evidence base is not in line with the views of these people, then they will be less willing to engage in evidence-based treatment plans.

The expert model, which can be perpetuated by the CAMHS practitioner him or herself, is a model whereby there is a belief that the person offering the help has superior knowledge, insight, and ideas about the issues in question. In this model, there is an idea that the person offering the help will be able to establish what the problem is, analyse the information, and suggest a solution to that problem. There is an assumption that the young person or family's interpretation of the difficulty is less valid than that of the CAMHS position.

If the clinician assumes the role of expert, the family will likely see him or her as in charge of the situation and in control of the agenda. They may believe this to be the best and most appropriate situation based on beliefs they hold about their position in relation to that of professionals. This can be compounded by poor mental health literacy.

The challenge with this is that the expert model can lead to the family only providing information they consider relevant to the problem and not taking ownership of the treatment. This can be disempowering and lead to a high refusal and drop-out rate and poor adherence to advice or treatment. The CAMHS practitioner needs to work at establishing a partnership model as a helpful, empowering, and productive approach. Working in partnership with the young person and family doesn't mean relying on poor mental health literacy. Instead, it is working with the young person and their family to present what the evidence says, and see how it applies to their lives and circumstances.

Most clinicians believe and say they want to work in partnership with young people and their families, whereas in fact they find this challenging. As with most organizations, bureaucracy and 'tasks' such as diagnosis, risk assessments, CAMHS assessments, and outcome measures can overwhelm the clinician, and detract from the reason they are there. In reality, some of the bureaucracy can be streamlined and most of the tasks form a natural part of the exploratory phase of a partnership relationship. Over time the information needed to complete the data quality requirements becomes engrained in the mind of the clinician, and is easily recalled when with families.

The families of children and young people with a mental health problem might feel they are being blamed for their child's problems or stigmatized by their contact with services. A benefit of the partnership approach to care in CAMHS is that young people and their families are more likely to engage and remain in relationship with the clinician. The key to this is the therapeutic relationship, regardless of the assessment and treatment modality used. Barriers need to be broken down. This can take many forms but it is important that the clinician remains authentic and true to their own personality and culture, at the same time as respecting and learning about the family's position. A more detailed exploration of these important issues can be found in the suggested further reading at the end of the chapter.

### Non-verbal communication

Non-verbal communication is a form of communication that uses wordless messages in the form of gestures, facial expressions, posture, eye contact, and body language. It can also include the intonation of a voice, the rhythm and style of speaking. Verbal communication is concerned with the words themselves – some suggest this refers only to the spoken word whereas others suggest it refers both to the spoken and the written word. From the first contact with the service, be that viewing the service website, service leaflets, referral letters, telephone conversations or a face-to-face meeting, the importance of developing the partnership and therapeutic relationship cannot be underestimated.

Forms of non-verbal communication include clothing, gender, status, social role, body language, and facial expressions to name but a few. A full exploration of non-verbal communication can be found in the literature but Argyle (1988) concluded that there are five primary functions of non-verbal bodily behaviour in human communication. These were to express emotions, to express interpersonal attitudes, to accompany speech in managing the cues of interaction between speakers and listeners, self-presentation of one's personality, and rituals.

Non-verbal communication interacts with verbal communication in a number of ways. Gestures can be used to strengthen a verbal message, but alternatively verbal and non-verbal messages can sometimes send conflict-ing messages. For example, a 5-year-old girl may put a toy from the clinic in her school bag. When her mother asks her if she has taken it, she might say 'no' but avoid eye contact, hide her bag, and fidget in her seat. Conflicting messages may be given during situations such as this but they could also arise from feelings of uncertainty, ambivalence or frustration. When mixed messages are observed during the course of the relationship, they can be highlighted to seek clarity and widen the exploration. In contrast, if the verbal and non-verbal communications complement each other, it could be used to highlight specific areas of the exploration. Accurate interpretation of messages is made easier when non-verbal and verbal communication complement each other.

Non-verbal communication is sometimes the only form of communication and people identify facial expressions, body movements, and body position-ing as corresponding with specific feelings and intentions. At times non-verbal communication does not effectively communicate a message, and verbal methods are used to enhance understanding. The CAMHS clinician will assess the meanings of non-verbal communication, as assumptions can be made that are not accurate.

Touch, pitch, and gesture are some things people use to convey what they would like to communicate, although they are not always conscious of it, as might be true of body movements and facial expressions. The qualities of a person's voice, such as volume, pitch, tempo, rhythm, articulation, reso-nance, nasality, and accent also ought to be considered. Some non-verbal communication from the helper can indicate to the young person that they are respected. This would include punctuality, attention and involvement, as well as holding the young person's gaze for an appropriate length of time, without being intrusive. Smiling, facial warmth, and pleasantness are also underrated in the helping relationship. They might be seen as wishy-washy and unimportant, but they are one of the foundations for building a helpful and open relationship.

## Verbal communication

Verbal communication is performed through words. The communicator tries to eliminate misunderstanding by putting across a message. Often we assume that our messages are clearly received and that because something is important and well known to us, it is important or well known to others too. This is also true in the helping relationship. If verbal communication is considered to include the written word, then it begins with the first letter sent to the family. CAMHS will attempt not to use standardized and impersonal letters because, although they serve a purpose, they do not do much to engage the family and give them a flavour of the service or the clinicians.

The use of interpreters is important when working with a family who do not have English as their first language. A disadvantage is that nuances of what is being said can be lost. Language helps us determine how we see and think about the world, so the use of interpreters is okay because limited language can restrict the thoughts of the people using it and the understanding of the person listening. The limits of the young person's or family's language become the limits of the information given.

Verbal communication has many functions and there are numerous ways of expressing ideas, goals, wants, and needs. It can be used to express what a person wants or needs, it can be regulatory, used to instruct somebody or maintain order. It is often an exchange, an interaction between people, and can also inform people of your intentions. It can be questioning, informative, cathartic, and exploratory.

Miscommunication can occur in the form of misunderstanding, non-understanding or misinterpretation. Verbal communication can be intentionally or unintentionally misleading. Words can support and encourage people; equally they can be devious, lies, and hurtful. Words can be used to avoid a subject or can be used to evoke specific beliefs, values, and emotions. The CAMHS practitioner has to be able to work with all these possibilities and many more when working with the young person and their family.

In the therapeutic relationship, the verbal and non-verbal communication of the families as well as that of the CAMHS practitioner is important. The CAMHS clinician should aim not to appear bored or inattentive, and frequently check the understanding of all parties. Many questions, both closed and open, will be asked to explore, clarify, and encourage the young person and family to be open and reveal what is troubling them.

### Other issues

For asylum seekers and refugees, particular attention needs to be paid to engagement and being sensitive to the cultural context and the needs relating to trauma. For example, it may be inappropriate to send out a team's standard first appointment letter inviting the whole family to attend and providing information about car parking spaces to an unaccompanied minor whose entire family has been killed and who is struggling to cope financially. CAMHS will attempt to consider who the recipient is of any letters and reports and adjust what is said accordingly.

## Questionnaires, outcome measures, and forms

Various tools have been developed to support the work of CAMHS. These assist in the diagnosis of children and young people, measure outcomes of their treatment, and generate data to show how effective the service is, and what developments might be considered. These tools range from highly validated and reliable tools to ones that have been developed locally for a specific purpose. Some of the commonly used ones are listed in Table 6.1.

**Table 6.1** Tools commonly used by CAMHS

| Tool | What difficulties does it consider? | What is it? | Age group | Who completes it/versions |
|---|---|---|---|---|
| Strengths and Difficulties Questionnaire (SDQ) | Emotional difficulties; conduct problems; inattention and hyperactivity; prosocial difficulties; peer relationships; total difficulties; impact of difficulties | A brief behavioural screening questionnaire | 3–16/ 17 years | Young person, parent, and teacher |
| Developmental and Well-Being Assessment (DAWBA) | All mental health disorders in childhood and adolescence | A package of interviews, questionnaires, and rating techniques designed to generate psychiatric diagnoses | 5–17 years | Young person, parent, and teacher |
| Health of the Nation Outcome Scale [Child and Adolescent] (HONOSCA) | The outcome of contact with mental health services | Five-point severity scales measuring 13 clinical features and parental understanding and local services | 3–18 years | Young person, parent, and teacher |
| Schedule for Affective Disorders and Schizophrenia for School-Age Children (present and lifetime) (K-SADS (PL)) | Affective disorders; psychotic disorders; anxiety disorders; behavioural disorders; substance abuse and other disorders | A semi-structured diagnostic interview with supplementary parts that, where indicated, look in more detail at specific difficulties | Under-18s | Interview the parent and child and gather information from other sources |

(continued)

**Table 6.1** Tools commonly used by CAMHS (*Continued*)

| Tool | What difficulties does it consider? | What is it? | Age group | Who completes it/versions |
|---|---|---|---|---|
| Conners Rating System | Hyperactivity; impulsivity; executive functioning; learning problems; peer relations; inattention | A comprehensive inventory of a young person's behaviours | 3–17 years | Young person, parent, and teacher |
| Screen for Child Anxiety Related Emotional Disorders (SCARED) | Anxiety and related disorders | Measures symptoms of childhood anxiety disorders | 8–18 years | Young person |
| Children's Obsessive Compulsive Inventory (CHOCI) | Obsessive compulsive disorder | The content and severity of symptoms | 9–17 years | Young person and parent |
| Child Revised Impact of Events Scale (CRIES) | Post-traumatic stress disorder | Monitors the re-experiencing of a traumatic event, avoidance of that event, and the feelings to which it gave rise | 8 years and above | Young person |
| The Mood and Feelings Questionnaire (MFQ) | Depression | Covers a broad range of affective, cognitive, and vegetative symptoms | 7–18 years | Young person and parent |
| CHASE | Experience of the service | Covers the main priorities for children and young people in relation to the practicalities, therapeutic process, and outcomes of CAMHS intervention | Reading age of 8 and above | Young person |

| Experience of Service Use Questionnaire (ESQ) (used to be called the CHI questionnaire) | Experience of the service | A mixture or rating scales and open questions | 0–18 years | Young person |
|---|---|---|---|---|
| Children's Global Assessment Scale (CGAS) | General functioning of a young person | A numeric scale (0 to 99) | 4–18 years | Clinician |
| Developmental Disability CGAS (DD-CGAS) | General functioning of a young person with a developmental disability | The same as the CGAS but young people with a developmental disability | 4–16 years | Clinician |
| Structured Assessment of Violence Risk in Youth (SAVRY) | Risk of violence to others | An aid to assessment | 12–18 years | Clinician |
| ERASOR | Risk of sexually harmful behaviour | An aid to assessment | 12–18 years | Clinician |
| DASH | Protective factors in relation to sexually harmful behaviour | An aid to assessment | 12–18 years | Clinician |
| Beck Youth Inventory | Depression, anxiety, anger disruptive behaviour, self-concept | Five self-report scales | 7–18 years | Young person |

Most tools have multiple purposes and can be used for screening, both as an outcome measure and for research. Some consider a specific disorder whereas others consider an aspect of the young person's behaviour or functioning. Some are for the young person to complete, others include versions for the young person, the parent, and the teacher to complete, whereas others are for the CAMHS clinician to complete.

These tools should never be considered to replace clinical judgement and experience. Instead, they should be used to inform the assessment, treatment and service design, and should only be used on the population they are validated for, unless the work is contributing to the validation of the tool for another population.

Young people and their families can often feel overwhelmed with pieces of paper to fill in and being asked the same questions repeatedly. CAMHS needs to bear this in mind. It is important that the use of tools is done in a thoughtful way, with developmentally appropriate explanations as to why and how they should be completed. Many of them are available online, and have been translated and validated for use in a number of languages; others have to be bought at significant cost to the local CAMHS.

A number of CAMHS are involved in the Child Outcomes Research Consortium (CORC), which aims to foster the effective and routine use of outcome measures in work with children and young people who experience mental health and emotional well-being difficulties. The services involved in this initiative use the same outcome measures and submit the data, without the young person being identifiable, to a central database. In return, they receive data back, showing how their local population and performance compare with other CAMHS nationally.

## Consent, capacity, and confidentiality

The issues surrounding consent, capacity, and confidentiality are often confusing and unhelpful to partner agencies and can lead to fractured working relationships if not explained and understood clearly. CAMHS, as with every service delivering healthcare, is bound by laws that govern the rights of the patient, although these laws are superseded by others, such as laws concerned with safeguarding and criminal activity, under specific circumstances.

---

**Box 6.1: The case of Jacob**

Jacob is a 15-year-old boy who has been referred to CAMHS by his head of year at school. The referral letter said that he had agreed to be referred to CAMHS but did not want his parents to find out. The referral letter explained that Jacob had missed school on a number of occasions and he was not engaging in his education. This was out of keeping with his character and usual behaviour.

At his initial assessment, Jacob was seen by a CAMHS nurse. During the assessment he engaged well and was clearly an intelligent young person, who could articulate well. He was clear that he did not want his parents to know that he was being seen by CAMHS because 'they have enough on their plate'.

Towards the end of the assessment, Jacob disclosed suicidal ideas. He had been thinking about ending his life and had stored paracetamol in his bedroom to use if he decided to follow through. He denied that he was planning to end his life now, but felt 'reassured' that the tablets were available if he needed them.

The legal framework in relation to confidentiality, consent, and capacity is set out below. Consider Jacob as you read. This section will end with an explanation of the appropriate action a CAMHS practitioner should take.

## Capacity and competence

The capacity to consent to treatment is usually established by a person's status as an adult in society and the legal age of capacity is 16. Competence is used to determine if a young person under the age of 16 is able to provide consent.

The Mental Capacity Act 2005 provides the framework for making decisions about capacity in relation to persons aged 16 or over who lack capacity to consent. It is decision-specific, relating to particular decisions at particular times. The Mental Capacity Act Code of Practice offers guidance on the key issues. If a person lacks capacity to consent to care and treatment, it can be provided if it is in the person's best interests but there are limits to this, such as the restriction of liberty (deprivation of liberty safeguards [DOLS]) and advance decisions.

The Family Reform Act 1987 gave 16- and 17-year-olds the right to consent to treatment as adults do. Gillick competency and the Fraser guidelines are used to decide whether a child or young person is mature enough to make decisions for themselves. The principles are taken from a case relating to contraception that was brought before the House of Lords.

Comments made by Lord Scarman in 1985 are used to test 'Gillick competency'. He said, 'It is not enough that she should understand the nature of the advice which is being given, she must also have a sufficient maturity to understand what is involved', and determined that 'Parental right yields to the child's right to make his own decisions when he reaches a sufficient understanding and intelligence to be capable of making up his own mind on the matter requiring decision.'

The Fraser guidelines relate to contraception but the principles have been applied to CAMHS. Principally, this is that the young person understands the advice, they cannot be persuaded to inform their parents about their health issues or involvement with health services, is likely to suffer physical or mental health difficulties if treatment or advice is not received, and that their best interests are being served. In cases where a young person is deemed 'Gillick competent' and refuses to consent to treatment, a court can overrule their decision if this could lead to death or severe permanent injury.

In order to determine if a child is competent enough to make a decision, they need to be able to understand information about the proposed treatment such as the purpose, risks and effects, chances of success, and any alternatives. The British Medical Association and Law Society (1999) recommend considering the young person's:

- ability to understand that there is a choice and that choices have consequences;
- willingness and ability to make a choice (including the option of choosing that someone else makes treatment decisions);
- understanding of the nature and purpose of the proposed procedure;
- understanding of the proposed procedure's risks and effects;
- understanding of alternatives to the procedure and the risks attached to them, and the consequences of no treatment; and
- freedom from pressure.

In relation to admission to hospital, a young person who is aged 16 or 17 cannot be detained solely on the consent of their parent(s). Similarly, a young person of 16 or 17 with capacity is able to consent to their admission even if their parents do not wish that to be the case.

## Consent

- Remember when you were 15 years old, when you had a difficulty or problem, who did you share it with and how much detail did you want your parents to know?
- Now imagine you are a parent and your child is distressed. How much information and involvement would you like in helping them address the problem?
- How would you reconcile these two positions?

For children and young people, the legal framework for consent comes from the Family Reform Act 1969, the Family Reform Act 1987, the Children Act 1989, the Mental Health Act 1983, the Crime and Disorder Act 1998, and case law. Knowing who has parental responsibility is important so that CAMHS can assess and treat the young person legally. Consent must be obtained before a health professional examines, treats or cares for a person. This consent must be voluntary and informed; it cannot be given under any form of duress or influence. Consent is an ongoing rather than a one-off event and the person who gives consent can change their mind and withdraw that consent at any time.

Assessment and treatment in CAMHS can proceed either with the consent of a young person or the person with parental responsibility, dependent on the circumstances set out below. Alternatively, the Mental Health Act 1983 may be used to treat people of any age.

1. *The young person has a person or persons who assume parental responsibility for them.* Treatment may proceed with the consent of one person having parental responsibility, even if there is opposition from another. The onus is on the person disagreeing to obtain a prohibited steps order. A mother automatically has parental responsibility for her child from birth. A father usually has parental responsibility. This is the case if he is married to the child's mother, listed on the birth certificate or has applied for parental responsibility and this has been granted.

   Same-sex partners who were civil partners at the time of the conception will both have parental responsibility. When the same-sex partners are not civil partners, the second parent can get parental responsibility by applying for parental responsibility or by becoming a civil partner of the other parent and making a parental responsibility agreement or jointly registering the birth.

   If the young person is the subject of a care order, the local authority has parental responsibility, which is shared with the parents. If the child is in care voluntarily, parental responsibility remains with the parents. There are others who can be granted parental responsibility, such as anyone granted a residence order or special guardianship order. Also, the local authority may rely on a protection order to acquire parental responsibility temporarily.

2. *Parental responsibility is forfeited once a child is given up for adoption.* Once a child is put up for adoption, parental responsibility is granted to the agency while placement is sought. When the child has been formally adopted, the adoptive parents take on parental responsibility.

As soon as a referral is received by CAMHS, two important questions will be asked:

- Who has parental responsibility, or is the child old enough to consent himself or herself? (Capacity and competence cannot be assessed until a clinician has seen the young person.)

- Has consent being given for the referral? (Are they aware that it has been made, why it has been made, what CAMHS is and agree to it?)

If the service is not assured that appropriate consent has been secured, by the right person, the referral will be referred back to the referrer for further clarification. Local services will differ in their approach to this. Some will telephone the referrer while others will send a letter asking for clarification. Either way, potential delays in assessment and treatment can occur as a result, so it is important for local CAMHS to communicate with potential referrers so that they are aware of this requirement.

Whether or not the young person needs to provide consent, it is good practice for the CAMHS clinician to work towards gaining consent from the young person. This will aid the clinician in gaining the trust and cooperation of a young person with emotional and behavioural problems. Without consent, avoidable challenges to engagement can arise. In addition, although a parent may consent, the young person may say they consent but actually be preoccupied with unconscious internal conflicts or caught up in a cycle of coercive behaviour with their parents, or have been victims of abuse. CAMHS clinicians need to work with the family and young person to ensure that consent is informed, legal, and not coerced.

Assessment and treatment should always be undertaken in partnership with the young person and their family. Whether or not they are competent, they need to be informed and involved as much as possible in treatment decisions. If they refuse, the objectives and treatment plan may need to be rethought, modified or delayed for more discussion. In addition, an independent advocate may be of assistance.

If no one with parental responsibility is willing to consent to a necessary treatment for a young person who is not competent to give consent, consideration is given by CAMHS to obtaining a specific issue order or asking the local authority to seek an order. This may lead to a safeguarding referral, as denying a child or young person the healthcare they require can be considered neglect.

Overruling the refusal of a child (competent or not) is only considered if discussion and modification of the treatment have been exhausted, the parents are in favour, and the child is more likely than not to suffer significant harm without treatment. In these circumstances, as when overruling the consent by a competent child, legal advice and a second opinion will be sought by CAMHS, a review date set, and the decisions recorded. Throughout all these considerations, it is important to note consent can be withdrawn at any time, as giving consent is an ongoing process.

## Confidentiality

Children and young people have the same right to confidentiality as adults. When able to make decisions about the use and disclosure of information they have provided in confidence, this should be respected just as it is with adults. The responsibility for maintaining confidentiality regarding privileged information provided by a young person lies with professionals who have access to it by virtue of their position. The Data Protection Act and the Caldicott Principles also require that reasonable steps are taken to ensure that information is only shared with those who need to know.

At their first appointment with CAMHS, the young person and their family are told that they have a right to confidentiality regarding information they disclose. At the same time, the exceptions to this are explained to them, such as when disclosure is considered in the public interest, where there are concerns about the welfare of a child, or it is required by order of a court of law. Confidential information is not the same as privileged information such as is disclosed to a barrister, and a breach of confidentiality is only made after careful consideration and if it is legal to do so. Whenever possible and appropriate, the young person will be made aware that this breach of confidence is to occur.

Public interest is taken to mean the interests of an individual, or groups of individuals or society as a whole. Specific measures to prevent crime, reduce the fear of crime, detect crime, protect vulnerable persons, maintain public safety, or divert young offenders may be in the public interest. Therefore, the health worker must, on a case-by-case basis, assess whether a disclosure is necessary to support action under the Crime and Disorder Act 1998, and if the public interest is of sufficient weight to override the presumption of confidentiality. In any event, the information must be processed fairly.

Where there are concerns about child abuse, clinicians follow the guidelines of the Department of Health, which state that 'the needs of the child must always be regarded as of first importance'. The ultimate responsibility to either disclose or withhold information in the public interest or the safety of the child lies with the individual worker. The clinician cannot delegate the decision, and cannot be required by a superior to disclose or withhold information against their will. Each health worker is responsible for their decision, and will be held accountable and must be able to justify that decision.

Breaches of confidentiality can be required by law or by an order of a court of law. Any confidential record may be subpoenaed as evidence in a court of law, including a coroner's court, investigations by the Health Service Commissioner or Mental Health Act Commissioners. The clinician may also be required to give oral evidence, if summoned, in addition to any records. Refusal to do so will place the worker in contempt of court and the legal consequences of such actions would apply.

In CAMHS, the young person has a right to expect that information given in confidence will be used only for the purpose for which it has been given and will not be released to others without consent. Where it is deemed appropriate to share information obtained in the course of the young person's assessment and treatment, CAMHS will ensure that before it is released that it is being imparted in strict professional confidence and for a specific purpose. Young people have a right to know the standards of confidentiality maintained by those providing their treatment, and these standards should be made known by the clinician at the first point of contact.

**Box 6.2: Jacob and CAMHS**

From the information given in the scenario about Jacob, CAMHS would need to decide whether he is competent to give consent to being seen by CAMHS without his parent's consent. This would usually involve a telephone call with the referrer during which the CAMHS practitioner would ask questions to ascertain competence. In this case, Jacob was thought to be competent and was invited for an appointment.

At this appointment, the CAMHS practitioner would assess competence as the interview went on. She would also be clear in her explanation of the limits of confidentiality early on in the appointment. Despite considering Jacob to be competent to make the decision not to involve his parents, the decision to maintain confidentiality would need to be reconsidered in light of the disclosure about having suicidal thoughts and paracetamol tablets.

The CAMHS practitioner would need to handle the situation with utmost care and sensitivity. Young people may give one reason they do not want their parents to know when the true reason is that they have been abused. The safety of the young person is the prime concern.

As the CAMHS practitioner explores Jacob's unique situation, she may decide to:

1. Discuss the situation with colleagues.
2. Tell Jacob that she is concerned about his safety and therefore a plan needs to be put in place to support him.
3. Put in place a safety plan with Jacob that has contingencies relating to his risks.
4. Decide the risk of harm from the parents to Jacob is too high and therefore a safeguarding referral is needed so that this can be explored further.
5. Work with Jacob to include his parents to put in place a safety and treatment plan deciding, with him, how much needs to be disclosed to his parents.
6. Override Jacob's wish for confidentiality due to the level of risk he poses and his refusal to give consent.

The plan will be placed under regular review and will be responsive to changes in circumstances. The level of confidentiality that is maintained will be fluid and respond to changes in Jacob's presentation but it is important, where possible, to maintain an open and honest relationship with Jacob throughout the process.

## Documentation

CAMHS keeps clinical records on every young person that they see. This is essential for the delivery of a high-quality service and supports the day-to-day care of the young person. Clinical records are a valuable resource because of the information they contain. This information is sensitive and personal to the young person, and so has to be managed appropriately. Good-quality record-keeping is linked with improvements in patient care, while poor standards contribute to poor quality care.

For CAMHS, it is important that the information in the clinical records is accurate, up to date, and recorded in the appropriate place so that it can be accessed easily when needed. Clinicians have a statutory obligation to maintain accurate records of events with young people and their families and to ensure that these are kept safe and secure. The terms of this come under the Public Records Acts 1958. In addition, CAMHS needs to be compliant with the NHS Record Management Code of Practice.

Each CAMHS should have a systematic and planned approach to record-keeping within their organization. This should include a strategy for collecting data about its patient population so that trends and service outcomes can be evaluated. There are legal requirements that must be considered and complied with to ensure that individuals' rights are respected. The Data Protection Act 1998 places statutory restrictions on the use of personal identifiable information including health information.

- In your view, what are the main responsibilities and requirements expected of all CAMHS practitioners?
- Why are these requirements important?

CAMHS records need to be kept up to date and it is the individual clinician's responsibility to do this in a timely and accurate manner. It should be recorded as near as possible to the time an event (e.g. an assessment, intervention or other action) was undertaken. The record should contain as a minimum, who is involved in the young person's care, an assessment, a care plan, a risk assessment and management plan, communications to the family and partner agencies, and a record of events. There should be evidence that the care plans and risk assessment and management plan are being reviewed regularly.

Any information about other family members or individuals involved should be documented in a third-party section of the clinical record. This is so that if the young person ever requests to see their notes, the information about other individuals can be removed. Despite that person not necessarily being the primary patient, CAMHS will still need to keep the information they have disclosed in confidence. In CAMHS, this is often the case when parents disclose that they have been abused as children. This may be one of a number of issues the parent does not want to tell their child, due to its sensitive nature. Their confidentiality needs to be respected and they, rightly, wish to protect their child from hearing information about them that might not be appropriate.

A helpful principle that CAMHS clinicians consider when writing clinical records is, if the young person were to present in an emergency to a clinician who had never seen them before, would that clinician be able to find and understand the information they need quickly and easily and will it make sense? In addition, any risks associated with the young person need to be highly visible.

Other principles also need to be adhered to. The information held in the clinical records must be adequate and relevant but not excessive, in relation to the purpose for which it is held, and must not be held longer than is necessary for that purpose. It should be made clear to the young person and their family that information received during the course of their involvement with CAMHS will be used for the purpose of the young person's care only.

There should be a restriction on secondary use of personal data received under any information-sharing arrangement, unless the consent of the disclosing party to that secondary use is sought. There is an increasing emphasis in healthcare services, including CAMHS, on building the evidence base. This may mean that young people and their family will be asked if they would be happy to be contacted if they met the criteria for a research project in the future. They may be identified as potential research participants through a word search of electronic records. The young person and their family have the right to decline, and their treatment ought not be affected in any way.

CAMHS will discuss as a team whether or not they need or should disclose sensitive information. There is always a preference to ask for consent. Generally a young person or their family are happy for this to take place if time is taken to explain why and to whom the information is being shared. Disclosure without consent can lead to fractured relationships and result in disengagement from the service.

If the consent of the young person and family is not sought, or is sought but withheld, consideration must be given to whether the personal information can be disclosed lawfully and fairly. CAMHS information is held under a duty of confidence, and can only be disclosed with the individual's consent or where there is overriding public interest or justification for doing so.

## Communication

CAMHS uses many forms of communication and local guidelines will be in place to ensure that these are conducted within the law, prioritizing the best interests of the young person. CAMHS practitioners will not email sensitive material or identifiable information about a young person unless it is via a secure email connection. Faxes can be sent if the recipient is standing by the fax machine and is able to verify that they have received the copy. Letters can only be copied to parties that the young person and their family agree to unless there are overriding reasons why confidentiality is breached. Telephone and informal conversations, as with all other forms of correspondence, are documented in the clinical records in chronological order.

Young people communicate in many different ways and CAMHS is catching up and adapting to these advances. Some services will offer a text appointment reminding service. Others will use email and texting as a means of offering an alternative therapeutic intervention. CAMHS needs to consider the sensitivity of the material being communicated when using these methods, and they should never be relied upon as the sole means of communication.

## Information-sharing

Information-sharing, or the reluctance to share information, can be the cause of much tension between CAMHS and partner agencies. This is often because each agency misunderstands the legal position of the other, or interprets the law in a different way. There is an obligation for all local authorities to commit themselves and partner agencies to local mechanisms that help remove barriers to sharing information and further put in place structures to support information governance arrangements. Some areas have chosen to put in place local information sharing agreements, which can sometimes be found on the local authority website.

Under certain circumstances there is a need to disclose personal information and data between agencies to ensure that the on-going care of a service user is not compromised. CAMHS must respect the young person's confidentiality. Confidentiality and consent are explored above, but there are circumstances under which confidential information may be disclosed, without consent. The grounds for breaching confidentiality need to be strong ones and a CAMHS clinician can override consent only if:

- a child is believed to be at serious risk of harm (safeguarding), or
- there is evidence of serious risk of harm to others or public safety (safety of others), or
- there is evidence of a serious health risk to an individual (public health risk), or
- the non-disclosure would significantly prejudice the prevention, detection or prosecution of a crime (crime), or
- instructed to do so by a court (court ordered).

### Safeguarding children

The Children Act 2004 places a duty on partner agencies to share information when it is in the best interests of the child. Section 10 places a duty of cooperation on all to improve well-being, and section 11 places a duty on partner agencies to have in place arrangements to safeguard and promote the welfare of children. These sections do not alter the way in which consent and confidentiality issues need to be considered.

### Offending behaviour

The Crime and Disorder Act 1998 sets out when people need to share information. CAMHS practitioners must be aware of this and are required to work within the law. Section 115 provides lawful power to exchange personal information if it 'is necessary or expedient to the successful implementation of the Act'. Although the Act does not impose a duty to disclose, agencies involved in information-sharing arrangements must decide the value and propriety of any particular disclosure for themselves. It is therefore important that CAMHS has information-sharing protocols between agencies that have been agreed and understood by both parties. When it is decided that information should be shared, this can be done with a chief officer of police, a police authority, local authorities, the probation service or health authority, even if they do not otherwise have the power.

Although section 115 ensures that lawful powers are available to all agencies for the disclosure of information to relevant authorities for the purposes of the Act, the law of confidence still applies to CAMHS. This means that anyone who is proposing to disclose information not publicly available and obtained through the clinical work with the young person and their family will need to establish whether there is an overriding justification for doing so. If not, it is still necessary to obtain the informed consent of the person who supplied the information. This is assessed on a case-by-case basis, and legal advice is sometimes sought by CAMHS if there is any doubt.

Multi-agency public protection arrangements (MAPPA) are in place to ensure the successful management of violent and sexual offenders and CAMHS is involved in these arrangements in some areas. MAPPA is not a statutory body but provides a way through which agencies can coordinate efforts to protect the public. Information shared through MAPPA is about individuals and enables partner agencies to work effectively to assess and manage the risks associated with these individuals. Case law has established that the duty of confidentiality can be overridden by the duty to prevent, detect, investigate or punish serious crime, or prevent abuse or serious harm.

### Safeguarding adults

Like children, adults can also be vulnerable and subject to abuse and neglect. Although less obvious than safeguarding children, safeguarding adults guidelines and legislation are relevant to CAMHS. Some young people with behavioural problems become very abusive towards adults in their life, and domestic violence in the form of physical and verbal aggression and bullying can be directed at an adult. This needs to be managed sensitively but local protocols and policies need to be followed.

**Key messages**

- Referral processes that are developed with partner agencies or where there has been good communication can reduce frustrations and foster good relationships between services.
- The laws that inform the young person's journey through CAMHS have developed over the years to protect the young person and the clinician as well as to maximize the chance of therapeutic engagement.
- Good communication and documentation are a key component in the care of young people.

## Further reading

Davis, H. and Day, C. (2010) *Working in Partnership with Parents* (2nd edn.). London: Pearson.

Harper, R. (2014) *Medical Treatment and the Law: Issues of Consent. The Protection of the Vulnerable: Children and Adults Lacking Capacity* (2nd edn.). Bristol: Family Law.

Wrycraft, N. (2015) Partnership working, in *Assessment and Care Planning in Mental Health Nursing*. Maidenhead: Open University Press.

# 7 Assessment in CAMHS

Children and young people rarely present to CAMHS with a single definable disorder. They usually present with a range of difficulties, and so an assessment by CAMHS is important. This chapter explores how thorough CAMHS assessments are, why specific areas are explored, the domains covered in the assessment, where the information is obtained from, and how diagnoses are made.

CAMHS assessments can vary in length and depth, from clinician to clinician and area to area. Some use an informal format, based on experience, whereas others use a semi-structured interview and standardized observations; others will use a combination of the two or different structures for different young people.

It can sometimes be difficult to understand why some areas, particularly sensitive information about a family's life, are enquired about in some depth, particularly if they appear to have no direct relevance to the presenting problem. A CAMHS clinician should never ask questions without a rationale, in relation to the assessment, for wanting to know the answer. Their rationale may be explained to the young person and their family.

Some clinicians use a set format whereas others prefer not to use one, but, either way, the areas covered should be similar. Assessments are completed by a clinician and rely on that clinician making subjective judgements based on the information they are able to gather and the observations they make. Teams with a specific remit, such as a forensic team or neurodevelopmental team, may consider additional areas of enquiry or place more emphasis on one area over another.

What is meant by diagnosis and why it is used in CAMHS are discussed in Chapter 6. It is acknowledged that time constraints and the pressure on services to reduce waiting times can mean that full assessments are sometimes replaced by shorter, more focussed or a triage-type assessment. Models for this have been developed, such as the Choice and Partnership Approach (CAPA). (These will not be covered in this chapter but further information can be found at www.CAPA.co.uk.)

It can be useful to have insight into what the difficulties might be prior to the first appointment, as referral letters vary in the quality of the information they provide. Some contain just one line, for example, 'I would be grateful for your opinion of this boy who has set fire to his house; his mother is understandably very concerned.' Others will include historical reports and a full description of the difficulties and the questions posed.

Often a clinician will be allocated to a young person due to their experience and expertise in a specific area of care. Information about this is obtained from the referral letter and any accompanying information. An appointment letter may be sent out with assessment tools, such as questionnaires, that the young person, their carer, and their teacher are asked to complete. Some services will use the Development and Well-Being Assessment (DAWBA) prior to seeing the young person and family.

The DAWBA is an online assessment tool, although it can be administered in person. It is completed by the young person, carer, and teacher who spend as much or as little time completing it as they feel is appropriate. It includes a range of questionnaires, free text options and rating scales, and considers the emotional, behavioural and hyperactivity disorders, without neglecting the less common but sometimes more severe disorders. (Further information can be found at http://www.dawba.com/.) This tool has a strong evidence base but can be very time-consuming, so most services prefer to use the Strengths and Difficulties Questionnaire (SDQ; Goodman, 1997), together with disorder-specific tools.

### The Strengths and Difficulties Questionnaire

Different versions of the SDQ are available for young people, parents, and teachers and can be accessed online in English and many other languages. The SDQ comprises five scales (emotional difficulties, conduct problems, inattention and hyperactivity, peer problems, and pro-social behaviour), and five statements per scale. For each statement, the respondent has to state whether it is not true, somewhat true or completely true. It allows a total difficulties score to be calculated (excluding the pro-social scale) and a score for each of the five scales.

In addition, there is an impact supplement question. The question about impact is only rated if the respondent answers 'yes' to the following question: 'Overall, do you think you have difficulties in one or more of the following areas: emotions, concentration, behaviour or being able to get on with other people?'

The score can be categorized as normal, borderline or abnormal using predetermined bands, according to normal, borderline or abnormal clinical significance, or can be used as a continuous variable. The impact supplement assesses whether difficulties upset or distress the young person and cause interference in their life, and can also be a continuous variable or classified into the same three bands. The SDQ algorithm was designed to identify three broad diagnostic categories, namely conduct disorders, emotional disorders, and hyperactivity disorders (Goodman et al., 2000).

Chapter 6 explored the therapeutic relationship and this is important to consider when undertaking a CAMHS assessment, as the assessment is an activity that is undertaken in partnership with the young person and their family. Together, the clinician will explore the available information and experience of the young person and their family and how it has led to the referral to CAMHS.

Time can be used more effectively in an assessment if information has been gathered and read prior to the appointment. This is not always possible due to the urgent nature of some assessment appointments and some parties being unresponsive to requests for information. The information sought may consist of documents such as school reports, social care reports, pre-sentence reports from the YOS, a statement of educational needs, education psychology reports, and previous CAMHS assessments. While reading and digesting this information, the clinician should keep in mind who the intended audience was, the purpose of the report, and issues that need to be clarified. They will be alert for conflicting stories and corroborating evidence for specific disorders.

Young people will often have divulged the same information about themselves to many people. It is important to verify the facts, gather information, and check it out with them. In addition, this can be a useful way of exploring their history and current difficulties. The CAMHS clinician will usually explain that they may need to repeat information but it is important that the young person is heard and their version of events and point of view are put across. Information from multiple sources can provide corroborating information or raise questions about the stories that follow young people and how they compare with reality or the young person's view of events.

In conclusion, when presented with a referral, CAMHS will note the concerns and presenting problems, as described by the referrer, but not treat this as the only version of events. The young person and the parents will have their own view of what the strengths are and what the problems are. The clinician will also come to their view of the situation. It is important for the CAMHS clinician to keep an open mind and explore both.

In general, a CAMHS assessment will include the following:

- Presenting problems
- Family history
- Social circumstances
- Developmental history
- Education and employment history
- Physical health history
- Psychiatric history
- Behavioural history
- Forensic history
- Substance use history
- Sexual history

- Personality
- Mental state examination
- Medical tests
- Formulation
- Diagnosis.

Risk assessment and management are also included in the assessment and will be covered in Chapter 8.

## Who is invited to the CAMHS assessment?

Some CAMHS will initially invite the young person and their family – either everyone in the household or just the parents – to the first assessment as standard practice, while others will individualize the invitation in response to the information gathered. Occasionally, the young person may be seen without the knowledge of their parents. This is discussed in Chapter 6, where consent, capacity, and confidentiality are considered.

It is sometimes unclear from the referral letter whether the adults in the household are the child's parents. It is important to know who the parents are, who has parental responsibility, and who the significant people are in a child's life. If the parents live separately, CAMHS need to meet, or if this is not possible for some reason, talk on the telephone with the parent who does not live with the child. This can sometimes mean contacting that person in another country. Their perspective of any difficulties and involvement in the treatment plan are as important as that of the resident parent.

Young people will be offered the opportunity to meet individually with the clinician, as will the adults. This gives each person the opportunity to tell their story and version of events without feeling inhibited by others in the room. The CAMHS clinician can then corroborate stories and identify areas that may be of concern that have not been spoken about.

Young people and their families can bring a friend or extended family member along to the appointment for support but the clinician will check throughout the appointment if the family are happy for them to be present and to hear the information divulged.

### Introductions

A CAMHS clinician needs to assess the young person within the context of their developmental age, taking into account the child's temperament, culture, and social circumstances, but before they do this, it is important that they establish a relationship with the people in the room.

All CAMHS assessments begin with everyone in the room introducing themselves, along with their role and relationship to the young person. Some CAMHS clinics have a one-way screen so that other clinicians can observe what is taking place. They will offer an alternative perspective from the clinician(s) present in the room during the clinical discussions. One or two clinicians may be present in the room. The young person and family should be introduced to everyone in the room and behind the screen. The reason for the use of the one-way screen should be given and consent obtained. The young person and their family will be given an opportunity to look behind the screen to satisfy their curiosity and for reassurance.

Following the introduction, the clinician will explain what CAMHS does and what its role is within the various services and in relation to the young person and their family. The clinician may ask the young person and other family members what they would like to be called and check the pronunciation. Before explaining what the assessment is for, the clinician may ask what the young person and the family believe the reason for the referral is and what their understanding of CAMHS is. The record-keeping policy within the local CAMHS will be explained, as will the opening hours and what to do if they need assistance in relation to mental health difficulties inside and outside office hours. This may be reiterated at the end of the assessment.

At the earliest opportunity, confidentiality and consent will be discussed and who has parental responsibility confirmed. The clinician will also ask if the young person or other family members are involved with other agencies that the family think could contribute to the assessment. Details of these partner agencies will be confirmed and who the family are happy for the assessment report to be shared with. This will be checked at the end of the assessment to determine whether specific elements need to be taken out for specific agencies. For example, a mother may be happy for the family GP and social care to know of her childhood abuse but not want the child's school to know. This is her information and she is entitled to have it shared in a manner she is happy with.

The family will be told the rules with regard to safeguarding concerns and disclosure of criminal activity. The young person will also be told about how and when confidential information will be shared with other people. Finally, the clinician will explain how long the appointment will take and what format it will take. The young person may be offered the opportunity to ask for a break if the assessment becomes too overwhelming.

## Presenting circumstances

During an assessment it is important to assess the way a young person views the world around them. Everyone takes in information, processes that information, and gives it a meaning. We construct a model of the world through this process. Then, through this construction, we anticipate situations and adapt to the world around us. Our models of the world, conscious or unconscious, are derived from our individual relationships and are unique to each person. During our lifetime, our constructs change through a process of testing and clarification and our social interactions are determined, in part, by the interplay of different social constructions. A CAMHS assessment usually begins with an exploration of the young person's view or construct of why they have been referred to the service and what the difficulties are.

Exploration of the problems begins at first assessment and continues throughout contact with CAMHS, even when setting goals, reviewing, and ending treatment. The exploration has to be undertaken in a tentative manner, without the CAMHS clinician taking control. Young people and families most often come to CAMHS to meet a perceived need, though occasionally they will be there because they were told it would be a good idea but do not know why. The family and young person are generally able to talk about their difficulties, although some may need prompting. The amount they disclose, how they disclose, and how comfortable they feel about doing so can be affected by many different variables.

The clinician will explore the young person's current functioning at home, at school and with peers, as well as their difficulties in functioning and reasons for the referral. Both the perspective of the young person and their family will be sought, as it is helpful to gain an understanding of what they would like from the referral. The answers to this inquiry are not always what the clinician presumes. It can also be different from the reason the referrer stated in the referral. The clinician may need to talk with the young person and their family about what the referrer has said and why they have made the referral, and may show them a copy of the referral for clarity.

Once the reason for the referral has been discussed, the clinician will start to explore the specific issues that have brought the young person to the clinic, as well as any other difficulties they might have. The perspective of everyone present will be sought and explored.

The clinician will ask a lot of questions about whether the young person has any worries, thoughts, images, feelings or ideas that bother them. This might involve a very detailed exploration of any suicidal thoughts and plans. Other questions might be specific to a disorder such as whether the young person checks things over and over again or washes their hands a lot more than most young people. There will be an exploration of the young person's diet, appetite, exercise, and sleep patterns, as well as any recent and sudden changes in them, such as reduced enjoyment of or participation in out-of-school activities.

## Immediate risk to self

When exploring why the young person has come to CAMHS for an assessment and what they want support with, the CAMHS clinician will explore whether the young person is at risk of harming themselves. They do this through direct and thorough questioning, rather than avoiding the subject. The young person may be relieved to be able to talk about their thoughts and feelings openly and honestly. A young person who is suicidal will usually try to let someone know of their plans, and they are more likely to share their feelings with friends of their own age or adults they know well. Self-harm is different and is often kept secret, even from friends and family. The person may feel so ashamed, guilty or bad that they cannot face talking about it.

The CAMHS clinician will try to gain a sense of the strength of intent the young person has of ending their life. When exploring these issues with a young person, the CAMHS clinician will ask the young person if they have ever thought about ending their life, and whether they have a strong wish not to be alive. They will be asked if they have made any plans to kill themselves and, if they have, what they are. The details of this will be explored by asking them a series of questions, such as: 'What kind of tablets? How many? Where would you get them? Where would you take them?'

The CAMHS clinician will explore what their ideas about being alive and being dead are and whether they have attempted suicide in the past. If they have, they will be asked to describe the attempt in as much detail as possible. Any young person who has attempted suicide needs to be taken seriously. An overdose may mean an immediate visit to the emergency department, as the harmful effects of tablets, such as paracetamol, can sometimes be delayed and even small amounts can be fatal.

## Family history

The family is an important area of the young person's life to consider in the assessment. Family members, both those the young person has contact with and those they do not, can contribute to the cause of the difficulties or be a protective factor, and are a key element of the treatment for most child and adolescent mental health problems. This can be in terms of biological and genetic factors as well as social and environmental factors.

While taking a family history, CAMHS often finds it helpful to draw a genogram (see Figure 7.1). Children and young people can become active participants in this process and are often interested to hear about their family. A genogram, which is similar to drawing a family tree, is a pictorial representation of the relationships between family members, and many of the areas that need to be explored in a CAMHS assessment can be addressed while completing a genogram.

In drawing a genogram, the symbols used have specific meanings; most are pretty standard but there are slight variations to these that have been adopted through custom and practice. A genogram should include a key at the side, so that the young person and their family can keep referring to their meanings (see Table 7.1).

The person referred can be represented by a bold outline or vivid colour so that they are quickly identified. A circle indicates a female and a square a male, while a triangle is used if the gender of the person is not known. If a symbol has a cross through it, it means the person has died. When the young person's parents have large extended families, a genogram can be drawn separately for each parent. Generally each generation is kept on the same

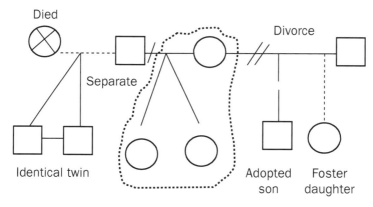

Died

Divorce

Separate

Identical twin

Adopted son

Foster daughter

**Figure 7.1** An example of a genogram is: Mother and non-identical twin girls living together, mother separated from the father

**Table 7.1** Symbols used to draw a genogram

| Symbol | Meaning |
|---|---|
| ☐ | Male |
| ○ | Female |
| —— | Connection |
| ------ | Living together |
| —#— | Divorced |
| ∕ | Separated |
| △ | Unknown gender, such as an unborn child |

line and siblings are drawn from oldest to youngest. Some clinicians put the name and age of the person in each symbol for ease of reference. Others will use a coloured pen to draw arrows indicating abuse from one member to another. A dotted line is drawn around groups of people who live together.

Key individuals within the family need to be considered in more depth than others. This will be because they are genetically very closely related, their living arrangements are closely linked or there is a significant amount of contact between the young person and particular family members. CAMHS needs to clarify whether 'aunts' and 'uncles' are indeed 'aunts' and 'uncles' or merely close family friends.

As the family's life and details are explored, CAMHS will try to ascertain how family members relate to one another, and whether there are patterns of mental health, physical health, abuse or substance misuse difficulties or criminality. Also, whether the family unit comprises biological relatives only, or whether someone has been fostered or adopted, or is a step-parent or step-child.

> Draw a genogram of your extended family. What are the stories and relationships that come to mind as you do this?

To understand who has an impact on the young person and what family narratives are at play, information is gathered about the social circumstances of the family and of each member, such as who lives with whom, what their work situations and educational backgrounds are, and any history of mental or physical health problems. Parenting styles and family belief systems will be explored, as will the family norms in relation to discipline and praise. The temperament of each person may also be considered or 'stories' about individuals.

At an appropriate time during the assessment, when a relationship between the clinician and family has been established, any issues of abuse, tension, antagonism, conflict or violence within the family can be addressed. These can be very difficult topics for families and need to be handled sensitively. The CAMHS clinician will explore positive and negative themes in relationships between adults within the young person's family, such as domestic violence and parental well-being, including their mental health, substance misuse (including whether alcohol or drugs were used during pregnancy), and criminal behaviour.

Some parents are unable to contain their personal experience of abuse and will talk freely, and inappropriately, in front of the children about it. It is the clinician's role to protect the child and provide the parent with time to talk on a one-to-one basis with the clinician. This may mean making another appointment in the future.

### Parenting styles

Rules are an important part of everyday life. They make it possible for young people to get along with one another and learn how to function in adulthood. If children do not learn how to behave, they will find it difficult to get on, both with grown-ups and with other children. They will find schoolwork difficult, will misbehave, and will probably become unhappy and frustrated. While exploring the family history, evidence of the positive and negative aspects of parenting, in particular, any use of coercive discipline, will be noted, as will the 'quality' of the parent–child relationship.

## Social circumstances

The CAMHS clinician will also explore the social circumstances of the young person and their family, including their accommodation and living conditions, how secure their housing is, whether the young person shares a bedroom, and, if so, who with. The family's financial position will also be addressed.

As the genogram begins to take shape, it may become apparent that there is a large extended family, and the clinician will explore how close they live from one another and whether they are able to provide practical and emotional support. This is important to explore because the behaviour and circumstances of the family may be a contributing factor to the problem being addressed or may impact ongoing care and treatment.

The clinician might ask the young person, if they were shipwrecked on a desert island and were allowed one person to be with them, who that person would be. This opens the door to explore the nature of different relationships and friendships.

### Religion and spirituality

Religious and spiritual affiliations can provide a young person and their family with much needed support and reassurance. Conversely, poor mental health literacy in religious communities can work against any treatment plans. Families may wish to compartmentalize their life and keep their mental health service involvement and religious affiliations separate, and this needs to be respected while leaving the door to future discussion open. While respecting the desires of the family, the CAMHS clinician will try to gain a better understanding of the young person's life. Involving spiritual leaders in any care plan can help with compliance.

### Culture

Concepts of mental illness and understanding of the origins of young people's mental, emotional, and behavioural difficulties vary greatly across cultures. In addition, the expression of these difficulties, both verbally and non-verbally, will vary enormously. Culture has a wide-ranging impact on the formulation of care plans, treatment, and outcomes for young people and should not be ignored.

Ethnicity is relevant because it provides an insight into the cultural experience of a young person. In addition, the effects and side-effects of some medications have been shown to vary across ethnic groups, yet this is rarely considered when prescribing medications. Expectations about the safety and effectiveness of any therapeutic intervention, whether that be medications or a psychological therapy, are shaped by the patient's sociocultural background and individual experience, so it is important to have open and transparent conversations about this from the outset.

### Asylum seekers and refugees

Asylum seekers and refugees are frequently referred to CAMHS because of the at times harrowing situations they will have experienced. If not already familiar with the young person's country of origin, the CAMHS clinician will find it very helpful to find out more about their country and culture before the first session. The clinician will explain that they are not part of the asylum-seeking process, and ensure that the young person understands the reason for the assessment.

The clinician may ask the young person about political, religious, racial or other affiliations that he or she believes relevant to the trauma experience and asylum process. Since interpreters are frequently used, the CAMHS clinician will attempt to find out about the young person's background beforehand if possible, as difficulties can arise when the interpreter is from the other side in a conflict.

In relation to an asylum claim, it is helpful if the clinician knows the asylum status of the young person and what stage of the process they are at. They will also want to know when the young person left their home country, when they arrived in the UK, how they made the journey, and who with.

### Friendship groups

Friendship groups are an important part of growing up. These allow a young person to experiment with conflict resolution and intimacy, and to share secrets, ideas, and dreams. Friendships and peer groups can also provide a challenge, particularly if bullying is involved, as it can have a detrimental effect on the bullied person's mental health.

The CAMHS clinician will ask a lot of detailed questions about the young person's friendships. They will seek to find out if he or she has a large group of friends and many acquaintances, a small, tight-knit group of friends, or a mixture of the two, and whether they are a leader or follower, as well as what role they take in their friendship groups. The clinician will try to gain an impression of the quality of these relationships and how that compares with accounts given by teachers and family members.

## Developmental history

CAMHS needs to have a good understanding of child development. In any assessment, the clinician will take a full developmental history. This will cover the usual milestones, such as toilet training, walking, and talking. Both the young person and their primary caregiver will be asked for their experience of the achievement of these tasks; primary caregivers could also be asked of their experience of achieving these tasks themselves. Some families struggle to give an accurate developmental history but the experience of growing up can be explored nonetheless.

The history will start from whether the child was a planned or unplanned pregnancy, the mother's experience of labour, whether the baby was breast-fed or bottle-fed, and how the parent and child bonded. If the primary caregiver had mental health problems at any stage of the development, this will be explored, as will any other significant events that may have had an impact on the child. In the same way, if there are unexplained delays in aspects of the child's development, the circumstances at that time will be explored and whether there were any investigations or interventions in relation to the delay.

## Education and employment history

A detailed history will be taken of the young person's educational experience, starting at nursery and how they responded to their initial separation from the primary caregiver. It is helpful to record year by year any specific strengths, difficulties, challenges or events. Permanent and temporary exclusions, including in-school exclusions, should be detailed, as well as any interventions put in place by the school to manage the young person's emotions and behaviour.

It is helpful for the CAMHS clinician to obtain the name and contact details of a member of education staff the young person is comfortable with and the family are happy for CAMHS to contact and liaise with. Where possible, school reports will be reviewed to highlight any patterns, such as poor concentration, or significant events. Also, education psychology reports, statements of educational needs, school action plans and school action plus plans, annual reports and attendance records can be informative. Some children and young people find a visual representation of their educational history (e.g. a life line with pictures, ages, and key works) helps them to engage in the discussion. Their current education details, needs and ambitions are considered, and any significant events in the near future, such as examinations.

Some young people may hold or have held a part-time job or be engaged in some form of employment. This will be explored and their current employment status noted. If a young person is not in employment, education or training (NEET), then CAMHS will explore the reasons why this might be and any barriers to change.

## Physical healthcare

People with mental health problems are known to have poorer outcomes in terms of physical healthcare. These physical health difficulties can be the cause of, an outcome of, or a contributing factor to the mental health problem. It is important that the CAMHS clinician considers the physical health of the young person. This is a very broad area and not all CAMHS clinicians will be expert, but a general screening assessment is possible. It is important to rule out any physical cause of emotional and behavioural problems. In a young child, this can be as simple as acute pain from untreated tooth decay that they are unable to express. Chronic and acute pain will make anyone, regardless of their age, feel low, grumpy, and agitated.

Height, weight, pulse, and blood pressure will be measured, offering a baseline against which future measures can be compared. Some young people will not have been to their primary care practice since seeing a health visitor before starting school, as they have never had cause to. Others will have been frequently for many different reasons. The clinician can explore the relationship with the GP, whether the young person is up to date with their vaccinations, and has seen a dentist and optician.

The clinician will explore the nature of any ongoing physical health problems or diagnosed conditions or illnesses and their symptoms. Serious illness or disability can cause a lot of work and stress in the family. A young person may also have been traumatized by a medical procedure they underwent. In addition, if there has been a delay in diagnosis or the future is uncertain, an illness can be very stressful. Following the diagnosis of a potentially serious or long-term illness, most young people and their families will need to adjust to the news and take time to come to terms with it.

It is important the CAMHS clinician find out if the young person has any known allergies. How a young person manages their symptoms and allergies can give the clinician insight into the child's life and how they are likely to engage with any treatment plans developed with them in CAMHS.

Consideration will be given to the child's pubertal status and whether there is any concern about growth or development. Another area of enquiry is in relation to head injuries. The CAMHS clinician will ask the young person if they have ever sustained a head injury or been hit on the head, regardless of whether they became unconscious or received medical attention. Traumatic brain injury in young people has been linked with offending behaviour and, in particular, violent offending.

## Psychiatric history

The CAMHS clinician will take a detailed history of mental health difficulties the young person has experienced previously and whether or not they had sought help. Information will also be gathered about previous assessments and treatments the young person and family have experienced, along with their view of the experience and what they felt was helpful and not helpful. If the treatment is ongoing, the clinician will explore this and request that they contact the therapist.

The clinician will want to know how any previous treatment ended and whether any recommendations were made for future work. At the end of the appointment, the clinician might request copies of previous assessments, care plans, and discharge summaries. The young person's experience of medication will be explored. This will include any previous prescriptions and any side-effects experienced, their compliance with the doses and timings, how helpful they were, and why they stopped taking them.

### Behavioural history

Detailed notes of any behavioural problems will be recorded, including patterns of negativistic, hostile or defiant behaviour, aggression towards people or animals, destruction of property, deceitfulness or theft, and serious violations of rules. The clinician will also note at what age these behaviours began, how frequently they occur, and who – if anybody – these behaviours were aimed at.

The young person will be asked about their emotional state, behaviour, and thought processes before, during, and after any incident and if they experienced feelings of empathy or remorse. The clinician will also explore what courses of action have already been tried and whether they were helpful or not. How consistently any behaviour strategy was applied by caregivers and teachers will be recorded, as well as any rewards for good behaviour and punishments for unwanted behaviour.

### Forensic history

A forensic history is a detailed account of the offences committed by a young person, regardless of whether they received a conviction, together with all convictions and court orders they have been subject to, and any involvement with the youth offending service. The CAMHS clinician might also enquire after the young person's attitude to the offending behaviour and to any victims of the crime, as well as their compliance with any previous or current court orders.

When considering the forensic history of a young person, the CAMHS clinician will record when the offending began, and whether there have been multiple offences of a single type or various, indiscriminate types of offending. The clinician will want to know if there were any direct or indirect victims of the crime, how old any victims were, and what relationship, if any, they had or have to the young person. The nature of the offence will be detailed – when and where it took place and whether the young person offended alone or as part of a group. Empathy and remorse will also be explored. Finally, the clinician might use a structured tool to assess any sexual or violent offences, as detailed in Chapter 6.

## Substance use history

Young people are less likely to be dependent on substances than adults but they may use substances recreationally, such as cannabis, or binge drink alcohol. The assessment will consider both illegal and legal highs, the frequency and quantity of use. The CAMHS clinician will ask what the young person experiences when they take these substances and what benefits and problems they experience as a result.

The clinician will wish to determine whether the young person takes substances in the company or others, when alone, or both, and how much they spend on and how they get their drugs. The CAMHS clinician may ask the young person to describe their relationship with their supplier and whether they are in debt to them.

## Sexual history

A sexual history is concerned with sex, sexuality, sexual abuse, and reproductive or sexual health. These can be difficult for young people to discuss and the CAMHS clinician needs to be sensitive to this. The clinician may agree to leave these topics to when the young person is seen individually. The clinician may agree not to include these details in the final report but will insist on raising concerns if safeguarding issues arise.

### Sex

If the young person is, or has been, sexually active, a detailed history of those relationships and their quality will be taken. The clinician will ask also when they had their first sexual encounter, and whether it was consensual and within the context of a relationship, together with the ages of any partners.

### Sexuality

Young people who are unsure of their sexuality or are lesbian, gay, bisexual or transsexual (LGBT) are more likely to experience discrimination, bullying and, as a result, mental health difficulties. A young person may not know yet what their sexuality is or they may not be ready to speak about it. The CAMHS clinician needs to handle this sensitively while being open to allowing the young person to change their mind or express uncertainty.

### Sexual abuse

During this part of the assessment, the clinician needs to take great in case the young person has been a victim of sexual abuse. Sexual abuse, in any form, can but does not always lead to mental health problems.

Sexual abuse does not just refer to penetrative sex; it also refers to things such as touching or exposure to material of a sexual nature. Young people who report that they are consenting to sexual activity are still being abused if they are underage. Female, male, and transgender young people can be involved in the commercial sex industry and it is important that this is viewed as abuse of the young person and an urgent safeguarding referral is made.

### Sexual and reproductive health

The CAMHS clinician will ask the young person about their sexual health and sexual heath checks, including their use of precautions against pregnancy and sexually transmitted diseases. Also, whether the young person is a parent or has aborted or miscarried a pregnancy. Any sexually transmitted infections will be noted along with how often they have been infected, whether they are a chronic, long-term concern, and which service they are receiving treatment from.

### Female genital mutilation

Female genital mutilation (FGM) is the cultural or religious phenomenon of the non-therapeutic cutting of a young female's genitalia and the associated trauma and damage – physically, mentally, sexually, and reproductively. The trauma associated with performing the FGM and of possibly being sent away or threatened with being sent away to have it done cannot be underestimated. When a CAMHS practitioner becomes aware of any threat or actual FGM, it becomes an urgent safeguarding matter.

## Personality

The CAMHS clinician will wish to find out about the young person's personality before the current difficulties. They will also ask about any changes in personality and when these occurred. The clinician might ask each family member to describe the young person's personality and temperament, or might ask the young person how they imagine specific people, such as a teacher, a friend or a parent, would describe them. They will then compare these views with what that young person actually says.

Not all cultures view a person's personality traits in the same way, that is, positively or negatively. The clinician might ask different people at the assessment what the young person's strengths are and what they like about them. Sometimes the family can find it difficult to say anything positive and the clinician will work to help them to vocalize something good.

## Mental state examination

All mental health professionals undertake mental state examinations even if they do not label them as such. A formal mental state examination offers the benefits of a structure, language, and form that can be used whenever the clinician is interacting with or observing a young person.

A mental state examination is a systematic appraisal, based on observation, of appearance, behaviour, demeanour, and mental function of an individual. It is always based on what is observed in the assessment and is an evaluation of mental functioning at a point in time, the point when the clinician sees the patient. It is based on professional judgement and the clinician's interpretation of the young person's verbal and non-verbal communication. Multiple mental state examinations over time can assist in revealing subtle changes to a young person's mental health.

It helps if the clinician is able to build a rapport with the young person, but it is not essential – what are essential are good observation skills. The clinician will interpret the meaning of the patient's verbal and non-verbal communication, bearing in mind what may be appropriate developmentally and culturally for that young person in the situation they find themselves. A mental health assessment is an abnormal situation and this needs to be kept in mind when commenting on a young person's mental state.

Key areas that need to be covered in a mental state examination include:

- Appearance
- Behaviour
- Mood and affect
- Speech
- Attention and concentration
- Perception
- Cognition
- Memory
- Insight.

Let us take each of these in turn.

### Appearance

To some extent, a person's appearance will provide an objective view of their mental state. This will be in relation to whether the young person is dressed in keeping with their age and culture, whether they are well groomed and adopt good hygiene, and if any distinctive features are recognizable.

### Behaviour

The clinician will detail the young person's behaviour in the room, including their facial expression, body language and gestures, posture, eye contact and rapport, and social engagement. In addition, a comment might be made about the young person's response to the assessment, their level of arousal (for example, calm or agitated), and any display of anxious or aggressive behaviour. Psychomotor activity and movement (e.g. hyperactivity, hypoactivity) and unusual features such as tremors, or slowed, repetitive, or involuntary movements will be noted.

## Mood and affect

Mood is the emotional experience of the young person over a more prolonged period of time. This is explored by asking questions about how the young person is feeling. The CAMHS clinician may ask them, 'What makes you sad, angry, happy or excited?' in order to get a sense of what the pervasive mood is and to measure it against what they are feeling that day. The clinician may also ask them what they would wish for if they had three wishes – this may give a sense of whether the young person has a sense of hope and optimism.

Affect is the immediate expression of emotion, observed in the assessment by the clinician. When observing the young person during the interview, the clinician will take note of the range of emotion that is displayed, for example, was the range restricted, blunted, flat or expansive? and was it appropriate, inappropriate or incongruous? Also of note will be how stable or labile the young person is, their level of irritability. The young person may be euphoric, elated, and full of optimism or have dysphoric mania where they are feeling high but also irritable, impatient, and agitated. A person with a stable mood is described as euthymic.

## Speech

The CAMHS clinician will observe the young person's rate, tone, and volume of speech as well as ease of conversation. During the course of the assessment the clinician will ask the young person questions and note whether there is any reciprocal conversation. Engagement in conversation will be encouraged by asking direct questions and follow-up questions, and be compared to how the rest of the family communicate. Reciprocal conversation may be commented on, although a young person asking an adult questions during an assessment would be unusual.

## Attention and concentration

Observations of the person's distractibility and performance on difficult tasks, such as completing questionnaires, will be noted down, as will their state of consciousness – that is, whether they are alert, drowsy or intoxicated, as well as their orientation to reality. This is often expressed as whether the person was orientated in time, place, person, and age.

### Perception

Anything that indicates abnormal perception will be recorded. There may be dissociative symptoms such as derealization (i.e. the feeling that the world or one's surroundings are not real) or depersonalization (i.e. the feeling of being detached from oneself). Hallucinations need to be differentiated from illusions. An illusion is when the person perceives things to be different from usual, but accepts that it is not real. A hallucination, on the other hand, is a form of perceptual disturbance where the experience is indistinguishable from reality on the part of the sufferer. It can affect all sensory modalities, although auditory hallucinations are the most common. In children it is common to experience self-talk or commentary as an internal 'voice', and care should be taken not to confuse the internal voice with a hallucination. It is important to note the degree of fear and distress associated with the hallucinations.

### Cognition

The content of the young person's cognitions and their thought process will be monitored. The content will note any delusions (a firmly held belief in something that is not real), overvalued ideas, preoccupations, depressive thoughts, and thoughts of self-harm, suicide, aggression or homicide. Obsessions and anxiety will also be explored. Unusual cognitive processes may be considered if there are highly irrelevant comments, frequent changes of topic, excessive vagueness, nonsense words, or pressured or halted speech.

### Memory

Memory is not usually tested formally unless a more detailed psychological assessment is being completed, but the clinician will be able to get a general idea of the young person's functioning, including their immediate, short-term, and long-term memory.

### Insight

Insight is more than knowing something is not right. It is the acknowledgement of a possible mental health problem, understanding the possible treatment options, and an ability to comply with these. When commenting on insight, it is important that the clinician does not pass on value judgements about what the 'correct' treatment is.

- Consider each aspect of the mental state examination and apply them to the last three encounters you have had with children and young people without mental health difficulties.
- Note the differences in each person and the judgements you make about what is 'normal' and what is 'abnormal'.
- Now consider any cultural dynamics that may be influencing either your interpretation or the young person's presentation.

## Medical tests

Sometimes, the CAMHS clinician will suggest that medical tests be carried out. Tests are usually ordered through the young person's GP or the local acute hospital. In some localities, arrangements are in place for work to be carried out in partnership with child health clinics. These tests are particularly important when evidence emerges during the assessment that there may be a medical component to the presentation, such as when the family report that the young person has fits or 'absences', or there is severe weight loss due to an eating disorder.

In addition to any tests that are ordered, it is good practice for the CAMHS clinician to measure the young person's height and weight. By doing this, changes over time can be noted and potential problems identified early. If there is a reported history of a head injury that has not previously been investigated, the clinician will suggest an MRI scan might be appropriate.

## Formulation

The formulation is a concise and clear summary of what has been learnt during the course of the assessment and a hypothesis for the reason the difficulties have occurred. This may be based on evidence from clinical trials, a theoretical framework, clinical experience or, most likely, a combination of the three. It is presented as an explanation or conceptualization of the information gathered during the assessment.

## Diagnosis

The assessment usually concludes with a diagnosis that is based on the information above, and is explored more fully in Chapter 8. As well as the diagnosis, differential diagnoses might be suggested. A differential diagnosis is a method where the clinician weighs the probability of one diagnosis against another. It is a systematic approach to identifying the multiple alternatives to the actual diagnosis that has been made.

## Ongoing assessment

Assessment is never definitive in CAMHS and is an ongoing process while the young person is being seen by CAMHS. The above provides an account of a comprehensive CAMHS assessment that is carried out when the young person is first seen. Children and young people develop, and the presentation changes over time. The assessing clinician may think it beneficial to gather further information or observe the young person in a different setting, such as at school, to gain further clarity about the diagnosis.

If the young person is found to have a mental health problem, a care plan will be developed (see the section on care planning in Chapter 11 for more details).

### Key messages

- A thorough mental health assessment lays the foundation for the therapeutic relationship and helps identify the most appropriate treatment for the young person's difficulties.
- Taking a thorough history across multiple domains enables a clear picture of the difficulties and their history to develop, even if the links are not clear to the young person and their family.
- A mental state examination describes how the CAMHS practitioner views the young person at that point in time.

### Further reading

Bellman, M., Byrne, O. and Sege, R. (2013) Developmental assessment of children, *British Medical Journal*, 346: e8687.

Goodman, R. and Scott, S. (2012) *Child and Adolescent Psychiatry* (3rd edn.). Chichester: Wiley-Blackwell.

Wrycraft, N. (2015) *Assessment and Care Planning in Mental Health Nursing*. Maidenhead: Open University Press.

### Useful website

For the Strengths and Difficulties Questionnaire and scoring system, [http://www.sdqinfo.com/py/sdqinfo/b0.py].

# 8 Specific mental health difficulties (Part 1)

This chapter will set out what diagnoses are and how they are categorized and labelled. A brief discussion will explore why CAMHS diagnoses young people and what advantages and disadvantages there are to this approach. The chapter then goes on to describe specific mental health disorders. The chapter does not address the need to consider culture and different cultures' specific ways of describing emotions and behaviours. A detailed discussion of culture and mental health can be found in *Aliens and Alienists*, a book by Lipsedge and Littlewood (1997). Other mental health disorders and co-morbidity (i.e. where more than one disorder is present at any one time) will be explored in Chapter 9.

## Diagnosis

To understand what a diagnosis is, the terms disease, sickness, syndrome, and illness need to be considered. *Disease* is a pathological condition recognized by indications agreed by practitioners, whereas *sickness* is the loss of capacity to fulfil social norms and *illness* is the subjective awareness of disturbance. A *syndrome* describes a group of symptoms that collectively indicate or characterize a disease, psychological disorder or other abnormal condition. *Diagnosis* is the name that is given to a group of signs and symptoms.

The process of making a diagnosis is to identify a disease or group of symptoms and allocate it a category. This is a subjective process but based on the best evidence available at the time of the assessment. Diagnosis is not purely a medical role. It is a means of communication using a set descriptor of symptoms and experiences that is helpful in ensuring that communication is in an agreed language. Diagnosis can be helpful in most cases. Most CAMHS clinicians engage in formulation and diagnosis, even if they do not see it as such. Failure to diagnose a child or young people can lead to a worse outcome for them.

The use of diagnosis is controversial in CAMHS. Some believe that diagnosis uses an elitist language that is based in the medical profession and one that children, young people, and their families will be unable to engage with. Those who hold these views often see diagnosis as a disease-based paradigm that adds nothing to the care and treatment of the individual.

They believe it only serves to strengthen the stigma that young people with mental health and behavioural problems may have experienced already.

A more positive view of diagnosis is that it is an agreed form of communication with a clear classification of symptoms that aid communication and the generation of evidence. It assists the young person and their family in researching their own solutions and aids in the selection of the most appropriate evidence base. Additional support and funding can often be successfully applied for if the difficulties are given a diagnostic label, and families and young people with a diagnosis in common can access support groups.

Some families think that a diagnosis won't help their child cope with their illness or symptoms, believing instead that it will alienate them, whereas others suggest that without a diagnosis, there is no clear idea of what is happening. There are some fears that a diagnosis will have a negative impact on future job prospects. Diagnosis is not an exact science and is not a standalone entity in CAMHS. It should always be coupled with a formulation, a helpful story of the young person's presentation.

Diagnosis is important but the concept of mental disorder is rather fuzzy and there is much debate about what CAMHS treats (DCSF/DoH, 2010). Usually young people are assessed and treated for disorders that meet the criteria for a mental disorder as defined under Axis I of the International Classification of Diseases, tenth revision (ICD-10; WHO, 1992) or the *Diagnostic and Statistical Manual of Mental Disorders V* (DSM V; APA, 2013). These disorders are 'a clinically recognisable set of symptoms or behaviours associated, in most cases, with considerable distress and substantial interference with personal functions' (WHO, 1992). This criterion was used by the report commissioned by the Office of National Statistics entitled 'Mental Health of Children and Adolescents in Great Britain 2004' (Green et al., 2005) and is used widely in research internationally.

What is clear to CAMHS is that mental disorder is not just about social deviance and conflict. The ICD-10 (WHO, 1992) defines most psychiatric disorders in terms of impact as well as symptoms. It explains that symptoms must result either in substantial distress for the child or significant impairment in the child's ability to fulfil normal role expectations in everyday life. Bird et al. (1990) explain that defining disorders solely in terms of symptoms results in high 'case-ness' rates, with most supposed cases not being significantly socially impaired by their symptoms, not appearing in need of treatment, and not corresponding to what clinicians would normally recognize as cases.

Children and young people do not always fit neatly into the categories laid out in the diagnostic manuals, and many will have been given different diagnoses from time to time. Diagnosis may be fluid and linked to the child's development and emerging signs, symptoms, and experiences. They may have more than one condition at any one time, labelled co-morbidity. Furthermore, when they present at CAMHS, their condition may be 'masked' by the use of substances. ICD-10 emphasizes that diagnosis is an iterative process and may very often change over time as clinical details emerge or developmental changes present themselves.

In UK CAMHS, the multi-axial system of diagnosis is used because it provides a clearer picture of the young person that can be used to formulate, communicate, and research. In the ICD-10 framework, freely available online, psychiatric conditions are classified by dividing them into discrete categories that are supposed to represent discrete entities, and are defined in terms of symptom patterns, course and outcome. The framework consists of six axes:

I.   Clinical psychiatric syndromes
II.  Specific disorders of development – includes speech and language, reading, spelling, and motor development
III. Intellectual level
IV.  Associated medical conditions
V.   Associated abnormal psychosocial conditions
VI.  Global social functioning.

## Axis I: Clinical psychiatric syndromes

Axis I covers the main mental disorders. It is possible to have multiple disorders listed under this axis such as depression and conduct disorder. Assumptions in relation to the cause of the disorder are avoided; instead, clinical features are elicited for description of the specific disorder. Although young people can have more than one axis in one diagnosis, there is a hierarchy of disorders as follows:

• Delirium
• Dementia
• Schizophrenia and other psychotic disorders
• Depression
• Anxiety and related disorders
• Personality disorders

The convention is that when more than one diagnosis is made, one takes precedence over the others. The guiding principles are that you start from the top of the hierarchy and work down. For example, when an organic mental disorder can account for symptoms, it pre-empts the diagnosis of any other disorder that could produce the same symptoms; and when a pervasive disorder, such as schizophrenia, has associated symptoms that are defining symptoms of a disorder lower down the hierarchy, then only the pervasive disorder is diagnosed.

## Axis II: Specific disorders of development

Specific learning disabilities are recorded under Axis II, including speech and language, reading, spelling, and motor development. Again these are descriptive and do not detail the cause. Developmental delay is not recorded here; this comes under Axis III.

### Axis III: Intellectual level

Axis III describes the current level of intellectual functioning and overall cognitive ability and is recorded descriptively. The cause is not included.

### Axis IV: Associated medical conditions

All health factors relevant to the mental health difficulty are recorded under this axis, including congenital syndromes and any past medical conditions 'of note'. Self-harm is also recorded here.

### Axis V: Associated abnormal psychosocial conditions

Axis IV provides a means of coding the young person's psychosocial situation where it is having an impact on their mental health. In addition, these psychosocial factors may be either a cause or an outcome. They can be present or historical and include a range of psychosocial hazards, from abnormal intra-familial relationships, such as physical or sexual abuse, to mental disorders in other family members, distorted intra-familial communication patterns, abnormal upbringing (e.g. in an institution), acute life events, and chronic interpersonal stress arising from difficulties at school.

### Axis VI: Global social functioning

Axis VI uses a 9-point dimensional scale, ranging from superior social functioning to profound and pervasive social disability. It reflects the patient's psychological, social, and occupational functioning and is rated at the time of the clinical assessment.

Let us now consider some specific mental health disorders encountered in CAMHS.

## Mood disorders

Mood disorders fall into three broad categories: depression, dysthymia, and bipolar affective disorder. Each affects a person's thoughts about how they see themselves, their life, and their situation.

**Depression**

The most common mood problem is depression, with a prevalence of 1–3 per cent in those aged under 18 years and is twice as common in girls than boys. Depression has distinct emotional, mental, and physical symptoms, characterized by persistent sadness, the inability to take pleasure in life, and irritability. The young person may describe feeling sad, hopeless or guilty, and having problems sleeping or eating.

Some subcultures within adolescence are preoccupied with thoughts of death or suicide, draw dark and negative images, and listen to song lyrics that are deep and intense. Involvement in these subcultures can hide the true depression that the young person is experiencing. It can also be difficult to decide if any difficulty getting up in the morning or difficulty studying is a normal part of adolescence. Although the young person may not use the same language as an adult to describe their feelings, it is important to ask them how they are feeling and hear what they have to say in their own words. Some clinicians find this a challenge because they are fearful that if they approach the subject of depression with a young person, it will upset them further.

There is a continuum upon which depression sits. At the mild end is an adjustment disorder that is a response to a distinct event. This usually resolves quickly during a period of 'watchful waiting' with the support of family and others. At the severe end, the young person can become psychotic and suicidal. Depression in adolescence is associated with a high risk for suicide and it is important that any mention of suicidal thoughts is taken seriously.

Children of all ages can experience depression. It can be hard to detect because the way children try to express it is usually different from that of an adult, and is often put down to understandable difficulties associated with their age or dismissed as part of adolescence (for example, a new school, exams, conflicts in friendships). Some young people present as shy, oppositional, grumpy or moody, and may report feeling physically unwell, saying they have a tummy ache, headache, or other aches and pains. Some find it difficult paying attention and ignore what people are saying, while others cry easily and frequently. Commonly they will lose interest in activities that they used to enjoy and will avoid going out with friends.

Young offenders in particular are frequently viewed as difficult and disruptive by the agencies involved in their care, and this may contribute to the non-health agencies not recognizing depression when present, and thus not referring on to CAMHS. As depression can manifest itself as anger in adolescents, it is difficult to see past the behavioural problems to see a young person who is significantly depressed.

Once a child or young person has been diagnosed with a depressive disorder, CAMHS will work with the young person and their family to put in place a management plan. This plan will include risk assessment and management (addressed in Chapter 10), as well as treatment. Treatment includes therapy, psycho-education, and medication. NICE (2005c) have published guidelines for depression in children and young people.

Depression frequently runs in families and parental depression needs to be considered when developing a treatment plan. A parent who is also depressed may find it difficult to motivate themselves to actively participate in any intervention or care plan. Work may need to be done in parallel, and with the consent of the parent it can be helpful if CAMHS and adult mental health services work together. In addition, consideration is given as to whether the child is acting as a young carer and in need of additional social support.

For mild depression, a period of 'watchful waiting' is beneficial as the difficulties may resolve. During this time, support from families, friends, and education staff will be helpful. Anti-depressant medication should not be used for the initial treatment. For moderate to severe depression, a combination of therapy, such as cognitive behavioural therapy (CBT) or interpersonal therapy (IPT), psycho-education, and anti-depressant medication is appropriate. The anti-depressants used might be selective serotonin reuptake inhibitors (SSRIs). It can take a few weeks for anti-depressants to start working and they should not be stopped suddenly. Some young people may be prescribed these for a number of years and should only stop taking them under the supervision of a doctor.

As with all medications, there are known side-effects of anti-depressants, some of which are serious. These risks need to be balanced against the risks associated with the depression and any decisions made after discussion with the young person and their family.

### Dysthymia

Dysthymia is a chronic low level of depression that lasts for at least two years. It leaves the young person less able to enjoy life, feel enthusiastic or ambitious. Dysthymia can continue throughout a person's life. The most appropriate treatment for dysthymia is the same as for depression.

### Bipolar affective disorder

Bipolar affective disorder, otherwise known as manic depression, is a mood disorder in which feelings, thoughts, behaviours, and perceptions are altered. There are episodes of severe and prolonged mania, depression or mixed episodes. A mixed episode has both manic and depressive symptoms. Children and young people with the disorder are more likely to have mixed episodes than adults with the same disorder. Bipolar affective disorder affects about 1 per cent of the population and is rarely diagnosed in CAMHS, although 20 per cent of adults with bipolar affective disorder report having had symptoms in adolescence.

Symptoms of mania include an abnormal, often expansive, and elevated mood lasting for at least one week. The young person will often act in a very silly way, be extremely happy, have a decreased need for sleep, racing thoughts, and thoughts that appear out of control. They will be observed to have rapid and often pressured speech. They may take risks and be reckless, and may become over-sexualized and have delusions of grandeur.

The young person's cognition might be affected, experiencing periods of confusion, or what is known as flight of ideas (excessive speech at a rapid rate that involves fragmented or unrelated ideas), and their thoughts might appear disorganized. This will often be coupled with them appearing frustrated, agitated, and quick to become angry or aggressive. They will sometimes have poor insight into their condition and make poor judgements.

Hypomania is a less severe form of mania, with shorter episodes of lower intensity. At times, severe mania or depression is accompanied by periods when the young person becomes psychotic (psychosis is discussed elsewhere in this chapter).

When having a depressive episode, the young person will feel very sad, guilty, and worthless. They will often be extreme in their eating or sleeping habits – too much or too little. They may complain about being in pain, have little energy, and lose interest in activities they usually enjoy. They may also be preoccupied with death or suicide.

The young person may lose friends as a result either of their lack of regard for others while experiencing a manic episode or because of withdrawing when depressed. This loss of social support during a period of their development when social networks are so crucial can have a significant impact. In older children and adolescents, there is an increased risk of suicide attempts. In addition, it can have an adverse effect at school, resulting in exclusion and rejection by peers.

There is no cure for bipolar affective disorder but effective treatment is available to manage the condition and aid recovery. It is important that treatment plans include an element of psycho-education for the young person, their family, and their school. Therapy to assist the young person to manage their thoughts, feelings, and behaviours may also be beneficial.

Different types of medications can be used and it may take time trialling different combinations to get the type, frequency, and dose right for each individual youngster. Some will need more than one type of medication. Medications are used to stabilize or maintain the mood, treat the depression, and treat the mania or associated difficulties.

## Anxiety and phobias

Anxiety has cognitive, psychological, and physical symptoms. It can make the young person afraid and panicky. They can become restless, tense and fidgety, and experience breathlessness and sweating. Some young people will complain of aches and pains or 'butterflies' in their stomach. It is unusual for these experiences to be present all the time but can be very distressing for both the young person and their family. Refusal to go to school is often associated with anxiety disorders.

The majority of children and young people who have this disorder have inherited a predisposition to anxiety, but trauma can also play a role in causing anxiety. There are different types of anxiety disorders, including phobias. Most are treated using cognitive behavioural therapy as the first line of treatment. Occasionally, medication such as an anti-depressant will be used in conjunction with the CBT.

Note that NICE guidelines for generalized anxiety disorder and panic disorders are not applicable to young people under 16, whereas the other anxiety-related guideline are applicable to this age group.

### Generalized anxiety disorder

A young person with generalized anxiety disorder will worry excessively about anything and everything, from the past, the present, and the future. This worry becomes so intense and all-consuming that it interferes with the young person's daily life. The excessive anxiety and worry will have been present for over six months. They may feel restless or on edge, become tired easily, have difficulty concentrating, be irritable, experience muscle tension and disturbed sleep.

Treatment includes education about the nature of anxiety, education about ways to identify, evaluate, and change anxious thoughts, and training in relaxation strategies. Positive 'self-talk' will be encouraged rather than negative self-talk. Families are encouraged to be involved in the treatment to reinforce and reward the young person using these strategies.

### Panic disorder

Panic disorder is characterized by unexpected and repeated periods of intense fear or discomfort associated with anxiety. These episodes are called 'panic attacks'' and can last a few minutes or hours at a time. They can develop without warning. Panic attacks are sometimes associated with other anxiety disorders.

### Separation anxiety disorder

Separation anxiety disorder is the excessive anxiety experienced by a child when separated from home or from a close family member to whom they are attached. Such anxiety is in excess of that which would be expected for a child at their stage of development. For a diagnosis of separation anxiety disorder, the fear and anxiety on separation and avoidance of separation need to have been present for a minimum of four weeks. Children with this disorder tend to come from close families and when separated from them they become socially withdrawn and sad and find it difficult to concentrate.

## Selective mutism

Selective mutism is an anxiety disorder that prevents children from speaking in certain social situations, such as at school or when with friends. These young people can often speak at home or when they are on their own but otherwise are unable to do so. They are not being oppositional, since the condition is related to anxiety and a fear of speaking and, as a result, some have conceptualized it as a phobia of speaking. Some children with selective mutism never speak, or are only able to say a few words or whisper.

Selective mutism is more common in females and ethnic minority populations with a prevalence of about one in 150 children. It is most frequently diagnosed in the first few years of primary school, as this is when it starts to interfere with learning but there is usually a history of people describing the child as shy and anxious prior to this. There is no evidence to suggest that the cause is related to abuse, neglect or trauma. These children can appear expressionless, unemotional, and may be socially isolated. Others may socialize only with a small, close group of peers.

The earlier a child with selective mutism is diagnosed and treated the better. Treatment normally focuses on the reduction of anxiety symptoms through developmentally appropriate cognitive behavioural therapy or play therapy. In addition, medications may be used to reduce the anxiety symptoms during any psychological intervention.

## Phobias

A phobia is an extreme fear resulting in the young person being very distressed and anxious. The fear has a significant impact on their lives. A young person can have a phobia of a specific thing, such as balloons, dogs or germs, or a perceived danger, such as with social phobia and agoraphobia. The earlier in its development that a phobia is treated, the better the outcome. Treatment usually involves CBT with exposure to what is feared.

### Social phobia

Social phobia is 'a persistent fear of one or more social or performance situations in which the person is exposed to unfamiliar people or to possible scrutiny by others' (APA, 2013). Social phobia is also known as social anxiety disorder and is the most common anxiety disorder in adolescence. Children with this disorder may have few friends, limited involvement in outside activities, somatic symptoms, and difficulty attending school.

### Agoraphobia

Agoraphobia is a fear of being in a position where escape might be difficult, or help will not be available if things go wrong. Leaving the home and going out in public can lead to intense anxiety. Young people with agoraphobia frequently also have a panic disorder.

# Enuresis and encopresis

The terms enuresis and encopresis are used to describe repeated incontinence of urine and faeces respectively. Some young people experience both, others just one form of incontinence. Often, when the encopresis is resolved in children who have both, the enuresis also resolves. These difficulties can have multiple components and causes. CAMHS may become involved in the assessment and treatment of these conditions when there is thought to be a psychological component. CAMHS works closely with child health clinics and GP practices as well as the education services and family to ensure there is a consistent approach to treatment and any associated physical difficulties are attended to.

Most children control their bowel before their bladder. The age by which children are expected to achieve continence varies across cultures, and the age of becoming continent varies from child to child. The most important thing is to start when that child is ready and not to pressure them. Children and young people of all ages can experience incontinence and it can be frightening, embarrassing, and humiliating.

## Enuresis

Enuresis is the recurrent involuntary passing of urine and can be nocturnal (bedwetting) or diurnal (any time of the day), primary (aged 5 or above and never been continent) or secondary (where a child has been continent for the past six months). The wetting may occur both at night and during the daytime in children who have previously been toilet trained. Some children wet the bed or themselves, whereas others urinate in inappropriate places even when a toilet is available.

Nocturnal enuresis is a distressing condition and can have a significant impact on a young person's emotions, behaviour, and social life. Rates of bedwetting more than two nights a week range from 8 per cent at $4\frac{1}{2}$ years to 1.5 per cent at $9\frac{1}{2}$ years years (Butler and Heron, 2008), although CAMHS can be involved in the assessment and treatment of young people with this condition up to the age of 18.

Children with nocturnal enuresis may have excessive nocturnal urine production, poor sleep arousal or a reduced bladder capacity. They may also have urinary urgency, frequency or incontinence during the day. It is important that physical difficulties are ruled out, such as a urinary tract infection.

NICE clinical guideline CG111 (NICE, 2010b) addresses nocturnal enuresis. Treatment is usually multi-modal and can include simple behavioural therapy with a reward system for remaining dry. Restricting fluids is not recommended but going to the toilet before bedtime is. Alarm training can be a helpful treatment for nocturnal enuresis and is most effective in the long term. A range of psychopharmacological drugs is also available, including desmopressin or imipramine. Most young people who do not have a serious neurological problem or learning difficulties can expect to achieve nocturnal continence sooner or later.

### Encopresis

Encopresis is the consistent soiling of faeces, in the clothing, despite previously having been toilet trained. The amount of soiling can vary greatly and there may be more than one cause. Initially, an assessment will ascertain whether a child has been adequately toilet trained. A medical examination will also be conducted to determine whether there are any underlying physical health reasons why the child may be incontinent. Although a diet high in fibre and fluids will help, a poor diet is rarely the sole cause of the problem. The young person may have developed poor toileting habits or have been toilet trained too early, making them very anxious.

Most children who soil themselves are severely constipated. They may have initially avoided the toilet, ignored the urge to go, and held onto the faeces as it was painful to go. Alternatively, they may have ignored their urge to go because they have previously been in trouble or embarrassed when they were either using the toilet appropriately and had an accident.

Holding onto faeces results in faecal impaction. This is when large, solid stools are stuck in the rectum and the surrounding muscles stretch and weaken. Watery stools from above the blockage then pass around it and appear as streaks in the children's underwear. If these streaks are not due to poor hygiene, the problem will usually get worse and an increasing amount of faeces will be found in the underwear.

There are no NICE guidelines specifically about encopresis, although some make reference to it, including the guidelines on constipation in children and young people (NICE, 2010a), when to suspect child maltreatment (NICE, 2009c), coeliac disease (NICE, 2009a), and urinary tract infection in children (NICE, 2007).

Treatment usually includes laxatives, toilet training, nutritional advice, and exercise. There may also be education for the young person and their families about the bowel, constipation, and toilet training. In some cases, a therapeutic intervention, such as narrative therapy (e.g. *Beating Sneaky Poo*;

White, 1968) can be of help. ERIC (Education and Resources for Improving Childhood Continence) offers support for families with continence problems, whether enuresis or encopresis.

## Obsessive-compulsive disorder

Obsessive-compulsive disorder (OCD) is a type of anxiety disorder, and young people with the disorder cannot stop worrying, no matter how much they want to. These worries frequently compel them to behave in certain ways over and over again. They can become preoccupied with whether something could be harmful, dangerous, wrong or dirty, whereas others worry that bad stuff could happen. Prevalence rates of OCD in children and young people vary from 0.5 to 4 per cent, and sufferers are usually diagnosed between the age of 7 and 13.

Obsessive-compulsive disorder is characterized by obsessions and compulsions. Obsessions are upsetting and disturbing thoughts or images that enter a young person's mind, which they find it hard to rid themselves of. These thoughts often become worse if they don't have or do things in a specific way. This then results in compulsions, which are a strong urge to do certain things. With OCD, there is an urge to appease these compulsions repeatedly and a fear that something terrible will happen if they are not done, and in the correct way. The obsessive thinking and rituals often take up more than an hour each day, cause distress, and interfere with daily activities.

Young people with OCD often find it very difficult to explain why they are doing their rituals, and may become more agitated the more they are pushed to explore it. Generally, their anxiety will lessen as they complete the rituals, making daily life difficult to manage. In addition, families can become increasingly frustrated and angry and this can lead to tension in the home.

Sometimes, the length of time it takes to leave the house increases to the point the young person is completely overwhelmed by their rituals. For others, the time they go to sleep becomes later and later as they have to complete so many rituals before going to bed. If the young person is unable to complete their rituals, they can become agitated and aggressive.

Young people with OCD frequently have low self-esteem and are embarrassed by their behaviour. In addition, they may have poor attention and concentration skills because they are concentrating on their intrusive thoughts. As a result, it can take a significant length of time for them to come to the notice of CAMHS and receive treatment.

There are many different types of obsessions that a young person may experience. These include, for example, the fear of contamination or germs, a need for symmetry, order, and precision, lucky or unlucky numbers, religious obsessions, sexual or aggressive thoughts, and a fear of harm coming to their family. Rituals include grooming, cleaning, hoarding, repeating, checking, touching, and counting.

Cognitive and psychometric tests can form part of the assessment and provide the baseline from which changes and the effectiveness of treatment are measured. NICE has developed guidelines for OCD (NICE, 2005a). Obsessive-compulsive disorder is a chronic but very treatable condition, and treatment can be multi-modal. Without treatment, OCD can become progressively worse, and have a significant impact on a young person's functioning and development. Cognitive behavioural therapy (CBT) is the primary means of young people learning about their OCD and anxiety. Occasionally, medication may be offered as part of the treatment package. Medication may reduce the anxiety enough for the young person to start therapy.

The CBT involves gradually exposing the young person to their fears, coming to an agreement that they will not perform their rituals, thus helping them recognize that their anxiety will eventually decrease and that nothing disastrous will occur. Sometimes treatment involves the young person giving the OCD a nickname and 'fighting back'. To fight back they may recruit an 'army' of relatives to battle with them. It is essential that the treatment is consistent and that it does not just involve talking about the rituals and fears, as this could worsen the symptoms.

## Traumatic stress, post-traumatic stress disorder, and abnormal grief reaction

### Traumatic stress

Children and young people will at times experience upset, reacting in many different ways and not necessarily immediately after the event. Normal reactions may be that they become clingy, have nightmares, start wetting the bed, and become more irritable. Most will adjust and manage, based on the support and reassurance of those around them.

### Post-traumatic stress disorder

Post-traumatic stress disorder (PTSD) is a delayed and/or protracted response to a stressful event or situation of an exceptionally threatening or catastrophic nature, which would likely cause great distress in almost anybody. About 25–30 per cent of adults or young people who have experienced a traumatic event will go on to develop PTSD. This event or situation could be a natural or man-made disaster, combat, a life-threatening illness, medical procedures, physical or sexual abuse, serious accidents, the violent death of others, rape, crime or even a young offender being traumatized by their own offending.

For a diagnosis of PTSD, there needs to have been exposure to a specific traumatic event and the persistent re-experiencing of that event through flashbacks or nightmares. This is coupled with psychological distress and anxiety. The young person may describe avoiding or be noticed to avoid places, activities, and cues that trigger the memory of the event. Symptoms can include hyperactivity, hypervigilance, sleep disturbance, outbursts of fear, panic or aggression, and psychological impairment, all of which have a negative impact on everyday life. There may also be an emotional detachment. The onset of these symptoms must be within six months of the event.

The NICE guideline on PTSD (NICE, 2005b) covers the whole life span but has sections specifically relating to young people. Trauma-focused CBT is usually recommended for children and young people with PTSD, and medications are not normally used. This form of CBT can last 8–12 sessions and is adapted to ensure that it is developmentally appropriate. A useful component of the treatment package is support and education for the family.

### Abnormal grief reaction

CAMHS will sometimes assess and treat a child or young person who is experiencing an abnormal grief reaction. The transition from a normal to an abnormal grief reaction can be slow and subtle. It can be difficult to determine what is normal and what is abnormal but grief may be abnormal if normal grieving is delayed, inhibited or prolonged, or if symptoms develop that are usually seen in the grief process and these replace or obscure the grief.

Treatment of the abnormal grief reaction will be determined by the symptoms that present but knowing the truth, talking about the death, and answering questions at an early stage, as well as being part of the cultural rituals, such as viewing the body (if they would like to), can help a child to adjust.

As time progresses, a child may start to worry because they can no longer remember the details of the person or 'picture' them. They may feel sad, angry, and anxious. When these feelings are unmanageable and present over a prolonged period, CAMHS can work with the child and family to support them through the adjustment.

## Medically unexplained physical symptoms and somatic disorders

Medically unexplained physical symptoms (MUPS) are when a young person suffers from physical symptoms for which no underlying physical cause can be found. The physical symptoms are inconsistent with or cannot be fully explained by a general medical condition. MUPS may also be referred to as a somatic or somatoform disorder.

Children will often express emotional distress by saying they are in pain. They might say they have a stomach ache or a headache. These usually pass and do not have a lasting effect on the child's functioning. Somatoform disorders represent the severe end of a continuum of somatic symptoms with some young people having epileptic-type fits or muscle weakness.

MUPS may be a symptom of another mental health problem or an expression of distress, sensitivity to pain or low self-esteem. Young sufferers will often miss a lot of school and withdraw to their bedrooms. They may have undergone numerous medical tests that may have been intrusive without finding a medical answer for what they are experiencing. This can cause great distress, with the young person feeling that no one believes them.

Treatment needs to be carefully coordinated between the GP, paediatrician, family, school, and CAMHS. The family need to be supported because seeing the child in distress and pain can be very upsetting. Treatment is best done with active participation from the family who may need to go against their natural instincts; for instance, the treatment plan might involve paying less attention to the symptoms while increasing the young person's involvement in social, physical, and educational activities.

# Eating disorders

NICE have developed an eating disorders pathway that addresses anorexia nervosa, bulimia nervosa, and atypical eating disorders, such as binge eating disorder. These address care across the lifespan. CAMHS is rarely the only agency involved in the care and treatment of young people with these disorders, and communication between services and joint planning is of utmost importance.

### Childhood-onset anorexia nervosa

Anorexia nervosa can develop from about 8 years of age, reaching a peak around 15–18 (Lask and Bryant-Waugh, 2013). In adolescent populations, the prevalence of anorexia is estimated to be 0.1–0.2 per cent, and is lower in younger children. Among adolescents, it is lower in males than females, with only 5–10 per cent of cases in males, while in younger male children the proportion may be up to a third. The mortality rate is 5–10 per cent.

The features of childhood-onset anorexia nervosa are as follows:

- failure to maintain weight or gain weight with age and development, or actual weight loss in relation to age (BMI < 7.5);
- determined food avoidance;
- abnormal concerns/preoccupation with weight and shape;
- amenorrhoea in post-menarcheal adolescents or delayed or arrested puberty.

Although a number of psychological and familial factors have been implicated as playing a role in the pathogenesis of anorexia nervosa, there is insufficient empirical evidence for these hypotheses. Cultural and social factors are also important. Generally, eating disorders are reported more frequently in societies where food is plentiful and thinness is valued. The risk of anorexia is high in young people who are involved in activities such as modelling and ballet dancing where there is an emphasis on slimness.

The onset is usually insidious and the most significant feature is food avoidance leading to severe weight loss. Patients are often secretive and adolescents are likely to avoid supervised meals such as school lunches. Distortions of body image are common, with denial of weight loss even when grossly underweight. Other associated symptoms include excessive physical activity in an attempt to lose weight and burn calories. Preoccupation with preparing food and feeding others is common. With decreasing weight the physical effects of starvation become evident. Patients complain of tiredness, lethargy, constipation, and cold extremities. It is important to bear in mind that in severe cases death may occur and use of the Mental Health Act or the Children Act may be needed, particularly when both the caregiver and the young person are refusing treatment and the situation is critical.

NICE (2004a) recommend that family interventions directly addressing the eating disorder should be offered. The benefits of inpatient care, in age-appropriate facilities, should be balanced against the effect on the young person's education and social needs. Dietary education and monitoring should highlight the nutrients necessary to support the child's development.

Multiple family therapy (MFT) is a recognized treatment that provides an intensive form of family intervention. It is usually delivered within regional, specialist eating disorder services. The aim of MFT is to help parents find ways of helping their child to overcome the eating problem. The families also attend groups with other families to talk about how the eating disorder has affected family life.

Young people with anorexia nervosa are sometimes admitted to a paediatric unit owing to medical complications resulting from extreme loss of weight. These admissions need to be planned and work needs to take place jointly between the CAMHS and the paediatric teams treating the young person. Some areas have treatment protocols in place to support this process.

**Bulimia nervosa**

Bulimia nervosa is rare below the age of 13 but becomes more common than anorexia by young adulthood (Lask and Bryant-Waugh, 2013), with the highest prevalence being among the 16–40 age group. As with anorexia nervosa, it is more common in females than males, although it is increasingly common in males. It is thought that 8 per cent of women will have bulimia at some stage during their lifetime.

Bulimia nervosa is an eating disorder characterized by episodes of binge eating, during which large amounts of food are consumed over short periods. Following a binge episode, the young person will purge their bodies through the use of laxatives and making themselves vomit.

The condition should not be diagnosed in patients with a diagnosis of anorexia nervosa, up to 50 per cent of whom also binge eat. Periods of binge eating are usually preceded by intense craving or preoccupation with food and intractable urges to overeat. Although fear of becoming fat and concerns about body weight are common, usually body weight is close to normal.

Patients usually describe loss of control over eating as the most significant problem. Up to 50 per cent vomit and binge eat or both on a daily basis. As this behaviour is associated with shame and guilt, self-induced vomiting is usually secretive. Disorders of mood are common, and include depression, guilt, and suicidal thoughts. Impulsiveness in the form of promiscuousness and shoplifting of food can also feature.

Most adolescents can be treated on an outpatient basis. CBT that has been adapted to suit the young person's age, circumstances, and level of development has been shown to be effective.

## Key messages

- Diagnosis is a method for describing a set of symptoms that are experienced or observed. It does not speak to the cause of the difficulties.
- Diagnosis can, when used appropriately, aid communication and enable the young person to receive the treatment with the best evidence base.
- Mood disorders can be experienced by children and young people but can have different features than in adulthood.
- Acting in partnership with child health practitioners, such as paediatricians, is essential when working with young people who have medically unexplained symptoms, enuresis, encopresis, and eating disorders.

## Further reading

Lipsedge, M. and Littlewood, R. (1997) *Aliens and Alienists: Ethnic Minorities and Psychiatry* (3rd edn). London: Routledge.

World Health Organization (WHO) (1996) *Multiaxial Classification of Child and Adolescent Psychiatric Disorders: The ICD-10 Classification of Mental and Behavioural Disorders in Children and Adolescents*. Cambridge: Cambridge University Press.

# 9 Specific mental health difficulties (Part 2)

This chapter follows on from the previous one and addresses psychosis, substance misuse, conduct disorder and oppositional defiant disorder, attention deficit and hyperactivity disorder, and other neurodevelopment difficulties. Finally, co-morbidity is explored, which is when more than one disorder is present at any one time.

## Psychosis

Psychosis is a group of disorders where the person typically perceives or interprets things differently from those around them – they lose touch with reality and become distressed and confused. Across the lifespan, the diagnostic subgroupings are schizophrenia (40 per cent), schizophreniform disorder (22 per cent), bipolar manic psychosis (17 per cent), schizoaffective disorder (12 per cent), psychotic depression (6 per cent), and delusional disorder (3 per cent). The peak age of onset is the late teenage years and early twenties with 20 per cent before age 20 and 5 per cent before age 16. Psychosis is very rare in childhood and so rarely seen in CAMHS.

Lay et al. (2000) found that at 10-year follow-up of those with adolescent-onset schizophrenia, 83 per cent had been hospitalized at least twice within those 10 years and 55 per cent more than three times. There was also a significant impact on the outcomes for this population, with 74 per cent per cent still receiving some form of psychiatric treatment, 57 per cent had a moderate vocational impairment, 66 per cent had a serious social disability, and 75 per cent were financially dependent. Psychotic illnesses are serious mental illnesses and 13.2 per cent of those diagnosed commit suicide; the rates for males are higher at 21.5 per cent (Krausz et al., 1995).

Early-onset psychosis is preceded by a prodromal phase of non-psychotic behavioural disturbance in about half of cases and can last 1–7 years. It can include externalizing behaviours and be misdiagnosed as attention deficit disorder or conduct disorder, leading to involvement in the youth justice system. Perceptual distortion, ideas of reference, and delusional mood can then begin to appear.

It is important for CAMHS to support those working with young people to recognize the symptoms and seek help from mental health services at the earliest opportunity. There is now considerable, if not consistent, evidence that the longer the gap between the emergence of psychosis and the initiation of effective treatment, the poorer the outcome, in both the short and long term.

NICE (2013b) have published guidelines on psychosis and schizophrenia in children and young people. A young person who is experiencing a psychotic episode may benefit from an inpatient admission to aid their assessment and to keep them safe. The treatment will usually involve medication that is a neuroleptic or anti-psychotic. The effects and side-effects of this medication will need to be monitored closely by CAMHS. Talking therapies, psycho-education, and work that is aimed at recovery will also form part of the care plan.

## Substance misuse

Experimentation with drugs and alcohol is sometimes seen as a normal part of the adolescent experience. Very few young people develop a dependency for a substance, although some go on to misuse. This rarely happens in isolation and a young person who is misusing substances is likely to have multiple co-existing difficulties, including social problems, mental health problems, and learning difficulties. Some groups of children and young people are particularly vulnerable. These include young offenders, looked-after children, young parents, those whose parents misuse substances, and those who exhibit oppositional behaviour.

Substance use, whether current or historical, should always form part of a mental health assessment, but there are conflicting opinions about whether CAMHS should assess and treat young people whose primary difficulty is substance misuse. As a result, the commissioning and service arrangement for young people who misuse substances varies throughout the country but, when CAMHS is commissioned, this forms part of a wider multi-agency service model.

When seen by CAMHS, young people will be asked about substance misuse. It is worth considering who is present when they are asked, since the answers may differ depending on who is in the room and who is asking the questions. The clinician will ask a young person whether they have ever used any substances, and, if so, what type, how they take it, how much, and how often. The young person may find it difficult to say how much they use, stating only how much it costs. The clinician will also ask whether they use it in company or alone. Finally, there will be a discussion about the impact on the young person's life and whether they would like help to kick the habit.

Most young people access services for substance misuse do so because of alcohol (37 per cent) or cannabis (53 per cent) use. These rarely require an addiction treatment programme. Instead, psychosocial, harm reduction, and family interventions are more appropriate. There are practice standards available for working with young people with substance misuse problems (Gilvarry et al., 2012).

# Conduct disorder and oppositional defiant disorder

All children and young people are at times naughty, disobedient, oppositional, and act out. They refuse to do as they are told, sulk, and test boundaries. This is a normal part of growing up. However, some young people have serious behavioural problems that last for a long time and impair their development and ability to lead a normal life.

Although not a diagnostic classification, some CAMHS clinicians will suggest that a young person may have an emerging personality disorder, particularly if the young person is 16 years of age or older. This may include young people with psychopathic, callous, and unemotional traits.

### Oppositional defiant disorder

It is not unusual for children to defy authority at times by disobeying or 'talking back' to adults but when this has been happening for more than 6 months and is more excessive than would be developmentally appropriate, the young person may be diagnosed with oppositional defiant disorder (ODD). This disorder is more common in children aged 10 years or younger; the other subtypes of conduct disorder are more common in those aged over 11 years of age. Estimates vary but are believed to be between 2 and 16 per cent of the pre-pubertal population with a higher prevalence in boys than girls.

A young person with ODD can come across to others as being uncooperative, defiant, hostile, and annoying. Their behaviour is directed specifically towards people in authority, disrupting daily life at home and at school. The young person may repeatedly throw temper tantrums, argue excessively with adults, and refuse to comply with requests and rules. They will deliberately try to annoy and upset others and blame others for their mistakes. These young people are often described as spiteful and vengeful, picking on people's vulnerabilities. Others may be offended by their obscene language, which is often with littered with profanities.

The young person will have repeatedly been told off, not achieved, and be excluded from activities as a result of their behaviour. This can lead them to have very low self-esteem and be moody. Although described as a behavioural problem, it is currently thought that ODD is caused by a combination of biological, genetic, and environmental factors.

### Conduct disorder

A conduct disorder is diagnosed when there is a serious behavioural and emotional problem that is characterized by a pattern of disruptive and aggressive behaviour and attitudes, violence and deceitfulness, as well as difficulty following rules. A conduct disorder can be socialized, unsocialized or confined to the family environment. There will be aggression and violence to animals or people, destruction of property, deceitfulness and lies, and serious violation of the rules.

Conduct disorder can occur in young people of all ages, but more is more likely to start in early life. The Office of National Statistics surveys of 1999 and 2004 reported that its prevalence was 5 per cent among children and young people aged 5–16 years. It has been identified as a strong predictor of serious and persistent offending and antisocial behaviour (Loeber et al., 2002).

The cause of a conduct disorder is probably multifaceted and includes genetic, environmental, psychological, and social factors. In relation to the biological risk factors, conduct problems and pro-social behaviour difficulties could have a genetic component. A low level of monoamine oxidase A (MAOA) is linked with conduct disorder, autistic traits, and criminal behaviour (Caspi et al., 2002; Kim-Cohen et al., 2006). Foley et al. (2004) found that genotypes associated with low MAOA increased the risk for conduct disorder only in the presence of an adverse child environment.

Young people with a conduct disorder may show aggressive, destructive or deceitful behaviours and violate rules. This may be demonstrated by aggressive behaviour towards people or animals, destruction of other people's property, lying, stealing, and playing truant from school.

NICE (2013a) have published guidelines on antisocial behaviour and conduct disorders in children and young people. Treatment is usually in the form of talking therapies and needs to be multi-systemic, involving the young person, their families, school, and community. Early intervention is important and the treatment plan may include cognitive behavioural therapy (CBT), family therapy, parenting programmes, multi-systemic therapy, treatment foster care, and dialectic behaviour therapy. Sometimes medication is used to treat other disorders that may also be present, or for the short-term management of aggressive behaviour.

Children with a conduct disorder may be irritable and have low self-esteem, and often throw temper tantrums. They tend to lack the insight of how their behaviour affects others. Young people who have a conduct disorder are more likely to underachieve at school, be socially isolated, misuse substances, and be involved in the youth justice system.

## Attention deficit hyperactivity disorder

Attention deficit hyperactivity disorder (ADHD), attention deficit disorder (ADD), and hyperkinetic disorder are all terms used to describe children, young people, and adults who have difficulties with concentration, impulsivity, hyperactivity, and attention. ADHD is the most common neurodevelopmental disorder of childhood with a prevalence of 3.6 per cent in boys and 0.9 per cent in girls aged 5–15 years in the UK, two-thirds of whom will continue to experience symptoms into adulthood (NICE, 2008b).

Although often considered to cause poor behaviour or problems at school, ADHD also has a significant impact upon family life, relationships with friends, school discipline, and society as a whole. ADHD is a clinically distinct neurobiological condition with the core behavioural features of inattention, impulsivity and hyperactivity, and care plans that are multi-faceted are used to treat the disorder.

The foundation of all helpful care plans is a thorough assessment of the difficulties that the young person and family are experiencing, and how they affect their lives. Information about inattention and hyperactivity alone is not enough to make a diagnosis; differential diagnoses need to be excluded. For example, there is some debate in the literature to suggest that PTSD, which can be characterized by difficulty concentrating, restlessness or irritability, and impulsivity, can be mistaken for ADHD (Weinstein et al., 2000; Yehuda, 2001).

Making a diagnosis is heavily dependent on parent and teacher reports, as no laboratory tests exist that can reliably predict ADHD. Instead, a comprehensive assessment is undertaken that includes a full developmental history, family history, physical examination, psychological testing, a review of school and medical records, completion of behaviour rating scales, and interviews with the family and child. Reports from multiple sources are essential and a school observation can be helpful. The young person, parents, and teachers may be asked to complete screening tests to support the information gathered during the assessment.

Treatment for ADHD should be multi-modal. This means a combination of treatments is used, such as psychological and educational interventions as well as psychopharmacological treatments. Medication should always be considered in consultation with the young person and their family, and their risks and benefits explained in a way that they understand so that an informed choice can be made. For most children and young people with ADHD, medication is an important part of treatment. Medications are not used to control behaviour or cure ADHD; they are used to make the symptoms of ADHD better.

Children and young people with ADHD are inattentive and have poor concentration, which can result in them taking their medication in a chaotic and inconsistent way. The family will often be a key component of the treatment plan, ensuring medication is taken correctly and reporting any effects and side-effects.

A number of different medications can be used. The first one to be tried (or the dosage) may not be the right one for a particular child. There may also be unacceptable side-effects. If this is the case, the dose can be adjusted or another medication tried. It can take a few weeks to find the right type, dose, and frequency for stimulant medication.

There are two main groups of medication that are used to treat ADHD: stimulant and non-stimulant medications. Stimulants stimulate the frontal parts of the brain that are not filtering out distractions as well as they should. The three most common types of stimulants used are methylphenidate, which is more commonly known as Concerta (slow-release form) or Ritalin (short-acting), amphetamine, and dextroamphetamine.

Non-stimulants are used when young people or their families do not want to use a stimulant, the young person does not do well with stimulants or experiences adverse side-effects. Atomoxetine is specifically approved for ADHD. It is not a stimulant, but it helps with inattention and with the hyperactive and impulsive symptoms of ADHD. It should not be used if the young person also has a depressive disorder, as the risk of suicide is increased with the use of this medication. The non-stimulant medication can take several weeks to reach its optimal dose.

Both stimulant and non-stimulant medications can have side-effects. Most are experienced when the medication is first used and tend not to last long. These may be a loss of appetite, headache, stomach ache, and sleep problems. A slowing of the rate of growth has been observed in some children and adolescents who take stimulants, but this has not been shown to affect final height.

Non-pharmacological interventions must be approached with the involvement of the family, young person, school, and CAMHS because consistency is important. Classrooms with a lot of visual stimulation may be very distracting for a child with ADHD and, particularly when taking tests or exams, the child may benefit from a room with minimal decoration and stimulation. Other therapeutic interventions might include CBT, group programmes, parenting programmes, social skills training, and psycho-education.

# Neurodevelopmental disorders

Neurodevelopmental disorders are disorders where there is an abnormality in the way the brain develops and works. Neurodevelopmental CAMHS teams usually see children and young people with a learning disability or an autism spectrum disorder plus another mental health problem.

### Learning disabilities

A learning disability is not a mental illness and so CAMHS will not treat a young person unless they also present with a mental health problem. A child or young person with a general learning disability finds it more difficult to learn, understand, and do things than others of the same age. The degree of disability varies considerably from mild to profound. These young people are more likely to develop mental health problems, in particular, ADHD, obsessive-compulsive disorder, and anxiety. They are also more likely to be on the autistic spectrum.

General learning disabilities must be distinguished from specific learning difficulties. Learning difficulties are when there is a difficulty in a defined area of learning but overall the child is developing within the normal range.

An example would be dyslexia. Learning disabilities are more general and there is no one cause. Some children may have the disability due to a genetic disorder and others due to an infection or brain injury, or damage sustained before or after birth.

Children with learning disabilities continue to progress and learn but more slowly than their peers. They will be aware of their surroundings but may not be able to communicate their thoughts and feelings. This can cause frustration particularly if the young person also has speech problems or is on the autistic spectrum. They may compare themselves to others and not understand why they are not able to do the things other people of their age can. Mental health problems are often overlooked.

**Autistic spectrum disorders**

Autism spectrum disorders (ASDs) are a group of disorders that affect approximately 1 per cent of children and young people, who have difficulties with their behaviour and communication. Asperger's syndrome falls within this group and is used to describe someone who has a higher level of functioning than others on the autism spectrum, and who has an intellectual ability in the average range and no delays in learning to talk.

People with an ASD struggle socially. There are impairments in social communication, social interaction, imagination, and flexible thinking. For a diagnosis of ASD to be made, there has to be evidence of an unusual development in the first three years of life. The nature of the difficulty will have a marked impact on family functioning and in most cases on education too.

**Treatment**

Treatment by CAMHS for mental health problems in a child with a neuro-developmental disorder usually involves an adapted version of the usual treatment plus support and psycho-education for families and other professionals involved in their care. The effectiveness of treatments needs to be monitored and the treatment adapted as necessary.

# Co-morbidity

Co-morbidity is the term used by CAMHS to describe when more than one Axis I disorder is present at any one time. There are numerous combinations and causes but the more Axis I diagnoses there are, the more complex the needs of the young person.

Some disorders are commonly associated with other disorders and, when combined, can increase the risk of a poor outcome. For example, conduct disorder is known to be a precursor to antisocial development, as is ADHD when it is combined with conduct disorder. Mordre et al. (2011) found that although combined conduct disorder and ADHD was strongly associated with later delinquency, ADHD on its own was not. In addition, ADHD is not predictive of re-offending, whereas the co-morbidity of oppositional defiant disorder/conduct disorder and ADHD is (Satterfield et al., 2007).

Co-morbidity could also be present when there is a behavioural problem, which then masks the emotional problem. For example, 'depression in adolescence can manifest itself as anger, which in turn is correlated with aggression' (Bailey, 2002); young people in this state are often diagnosed with a conduct disorder alone and their depression is not recognized. This could add to the young person's sense of worthlessness and hopelessness.

Some disorders are commonly seen alongside neurodevelopmental disorders. For example, obsessive-compulsive disorder is common in young people with Tourette's syndrome or tic disorders. It is also common in young people with other anxiety disorders, depression, attention deficit hyperactivity disorder, learning disorders, and trichotillomania (compulsive hair pulling).

## Key messages

- Children and young people can experience serious mental health problems.
- Behavioural difficulties in children and young people are not just the result of 'bad parenting' or children just being 'naughty' or 'bad'.
- Co-morbidity is not uncommon.

## Further reading

Kalid, K. (2013) *A Practical Guide to Mental Health Problems in Children with Autistic Spectrum: It's Not Just Their Autism!* London: Jessica Kingsley.

# 10 Risk

This chapter addresses the important area of risk and risk management in CAMHS. There are sections on safeguarding children and adults, the roles and responsibilities of CAMHS, as well as risk from and to others. Finally, risk management is addressed and how CAMHS learns lessons from serious incidents.

First, however, it is important to establish what risk assessment involves and what CAMHS needs to consider in understanding and making judgements about risk. Risk factors can be considered across a range of domains but can be theoretically divided into historical risk factors, social and contextual risk factors, and individual risk factors. For a complete picture of the risk profile, the protective factors are always considered as part of the risk assessment.

Risk assessment is a dynamic process and someone who is at a high risk at one point in time could present at a low or medium level of risk at another. Historical risk factors are static and largely will be unchanged, whereas the other domains are dynamic and change over time. When reporting or reading a risk assessment, it is important that it is viewed as the assessment of risk at that point in time.

Risk assessment can also take the form of a clinical assessment or an actuarial assessment. A clinical assessment is diagnostic and relies on professional judgement. It is intuitive and based on reviews of records and in-depth interviews. The benefits are that it focuses on the individual and explains behaviour, and can identify risk factors that are changeable and thereby inform interventions. The pitfalls are that it is not reliable or accurate because it is subjective.

In contrast, an actuarial assessment relies on statistical calculations of probability, based on data from large-scale studies. An actuarial assessment identifies factors that statistically relate to risk. The benefits are that it is accurate and reliable, and it identifies historical and demographic risk factors that are easy to identify. The pitfalls are that it does not fully represent the individual and their circumstances, or accurately predict behaviours that occur only rarely (e.g. serious violent or sexual assaults). An actuarial risk assessment does not explain behaviour or take into account positive changes or protective factors. It relies heavily on historical information.

A combination of actuarial assessment of probability based on established static risk factors and detailed clinical assessment based on research knowledge of dynamic risk factors enhances accuracy and consistency. A combined approach can provide valuable information to help guide interventions.

Risk assessment should be completed in partnership with, and communicated to, the young person and their family. In addition, information should be gathered from as many sources as possible so that the evidence can be corroborated. Sources may include school reports, local authority files, convictions, and interviews with the young person, family members, and professionals. Where information is lacking, this will be highlighted in the risk assessment as needing to be found at the earliest opportunity.

A CAMHS practitioner has to keep in mind that, as the assessor, their own experiences and constructs have an impact on their view of risk. Their view will be influenced by experience, values derived from family influences, education, culture, parenthood and being parented, one's own ideals, professional training, professional and social values, legislative duties and government guidance. Supervision and discussion with colleagues about risk assessments, formulation, and plans are of utmost importance.

When considering risk, the CAMHS clinician also needs to consider the resilience of the young person. Resilience emphasizes the skills and capacities that facilitate successful negotiation of high-risk environments, whereas working with risk alone will emphasize removing or avoiding factors that have unwanted outcomes. Although resilience is considered in CAMHS, a risk assessment is usually carried out with every young person. Additional considerations are the level of concern expressed by the family or other carers, other agencies, and the young person.

## Safeguarding children

Safeguarding children involves all agencies working with children, young people, and their families. They all need to take reasonable steps to ensure that the risk of harm to a child is minimized. If there are concerns about children and young people's welfare, all agencies must take all appropriate action to address those concerns, working to agreed local policies and procedures in full partnership with other local agencies.

The welfare of children and young people is crucial to the well-being of future generations, and the consequences of abuse and neglect can cause long-lasting damage into adulthood. Child abuse and neglect during early childhood have been shown to negatively affect early brain development and can have serious repercussions. CAMHS is frequently involved with children for whom there are safeguarding concerns and will often identify circumstances where abuse or neglect might be taking place. Many of the inquiries into child deaths and serious incidents involving children have demonstrated failings in the identification and sharing of concerns about safeguarding issues by the agencies involved.

Working with children to identify and manage safeguarding concerns and making referrals can be stressful, distressing, and demanding. In CAMHS there will always be someone, usually a named nurse and a named doctor, who can be approached for a consultation, advice, and support. In addition, effective supervision is important for promoting good standards of practice and supporting individuals.

CAMHS clinicians have the same responsibility as other clinicians to help ensure that children are safe from harm. They have a duty to identify signs that a child may be at risk and to take action if there is a need for protective measures. CAMHS will report any suspicions of risk to the appropriate authorities and do this consistently within the framework of legislation, policies, and procedures. They also must record and report any information that is available to them.

A child can be ill treated physically, mentally or sexually. This can involve the impairment of the child's physical or mental health, as well as their physical, intellectual, emotional, social or behavioural development. It is the responsibility of CAMHS to refer concerns to social care; they will then assess the situation and determine if action needs to be taken to protect the child. CAMHS has a duty to work in partnership with other agencies to safeguard children.

### Neglect

Neglect can occur whether or not it is intended on the part of caregivers. It can include the child not being stimulated or responded to, not being looked after or fed properly. They may be dirty or hungry. Neglect also includes not being helped with schoolwork or being supported in social activities. There may be a restriction of opportunities for learning and development. Most parents with a depressive illness will not neglect their children but some will due to their lack of motivation and energy. They may also be absent emotionally and less likely to pick up on their children's cues. A child with a mentally ill parent may be a young carer.

### Emotional abuse

Emotional abuse refers to the relationship between the abuser and the child rather than to an event or a series of repeated events that have occurred within the carer–child relationship. The interactions of concern pervade or characterize the relationship, meaning that they will be observed at different times and in different settings. The interactions are actually or potentially harmful. Emotional abuse includes omission as well as active abuse. Emotional abuse and neglect do not require any physical contact between abuser and child.

The example given under neglect above, where the parent is unresponsive and emotionally neglectful towards the child, would be considered emotional abuse. In this case, the parent may be preoccupied with his or her own particular difficulties and unable rather than unwilling to respond to the child's emotional needs.

An alternative form of emotional abuse is when the child is perceived as not deserving parental attention. In such a relationship, the parent will be hostile to, punish, denigrate, reject, and scapegoat the child. CAMHS sometimes observes developmentally inappropriate or inconsistent interactions with the child. Also, this may be an issue with parents whose expectation of the child is beyond or below his or her developmental capabilities. In both circumstances, emotional abuse is occurring.

The child may be exposed to confusing or traumatic events or interactions, such as domestic violence and parental suicide attempts. Even when this is within the context of a parent's own childhood experiences, it is important that the child's needs are the primary concern. Failure to recognize or acknowledge the child's individuality and psychological boundary would be of significant concern.

Another area of concern is where the parent uses the child to fulfil their psychological needs and there is an inability to distinguish between the child's reality and the adult's beliefs and wishes. Fabricated illness is a form of emotional abuse that can lead to physical abuse.

Every child needs to learn and have the opportunity to socialize. Failure to promote the child's socialization or to actively promote abnormal or anti-social ways of adapting, including failure to provide adequate stimulation and opportunities for learning, or involving children in criminal activities, is a form of emotional abuse.

There is a complex relationship between the age of the child and how severe the effect of any maltreatment is. An early onset of abuse is likely to interfere with the formation of secure attachments, and be associated with long-term maltreatment, unless there is early effective intervention. Conversely, a later onset suggests the possibility of previously established secure attachments and a shorter duration.

## Physical abuse

Physical abuse means physically harming a child, including hitting and shaking. CAMHS clinicians sometimes encounter physical abuse when asking families about how they reinforce boundaries and punish bad behaviour. The clinician needs to be clear that cultural explanations are not a satisfactory explanation, and any case of harm being caused to a young person will be treated as a safeguarding issue and referred appropriately.

## Sexual abuse

Sexual abuse involves forcing or enticing a young person to take part in sexual activities, whether or not the child is aware of what is happening.

The activities may involve physical contact, such as penetrative or non-penetrative acts. They may also include non-contact activities, such as involving children in the production of sexual images, watching sexual activities, encouraging children to behave in sexually inappropriate ways, and grooming.

CAMHS clinicians sometimes hear of a parent's experience of abuse at the hands of someone they are still in contact with, such as the child's grandfather. Despite not being directly about the young person who was referred to CAMHS, the clinician will need to report this historical information to social care in order to ensure that the young person is not at risk of abuse by the same abuser. Even if a parent doesn't want such facts to be reported, the clinician has an overriding duty to protect any child from potential abuse.

### Safeguarding processes

Each locality will have its own safeguarding procedures, policies, and protocols, which the local CAMHS will have signed up to. Every CAMHS clinician will have completed regular safeguarding training and be familiar with the safeguarding protocols.

## Risk from others and external events

Contextual factors also need to be considered in a risk assessment. For example, is the young person a victim of gang crime or are they living in a community where there is a high crime rate and culture of violence? Is there domestic violence at home or has the young person been exposed to war, torture or violence?

### Being bullied

Bullying occurs when one person picks on another repeatedly. The bullying can be verbal, physical, emotional or sexual, and the victim often finds it hard to defend themselves. Bullying increases the risk of mental health problems, including depression and anxiety, as well as the risk of deliberate self-harm and suicide.

### Community violence

Community violence and the presence of local gangs can put the young person at risk. Having a supportive family, community, and peer environment will contribute to the young person's resilience (Olsson et al., 2003), but it is clear that not all peer environments and communities are positive experiences. Young people are social beings and although it is generally thought that social relationships are positive and protective, there are some groups that can negatively influence or affect the young person.

Some children become fearful of leaving the home if there are gangs or violence in the local community. They may refuse to go to school and become anxious, a frequent response to the threat they perceive or have experienced. (Gang membership is considered later in this chapter.)

## Domestic violence and abuse

The definition of domestic violence adopted by the UK government is 'Any incident of threatening behaviour, violence or abuse (psychological, physical, sexual, financial or emotional) between adults who are or have been intimate partners or family members, regardless of gender or sexuality.' It includes honour-based violence, female genital mutilation, and forced marriage. Domestic violence and abuse are a cause of harm to children and young people of any age and create a significant risk in terms of mental health difficulties.

It is very upsetting for young people and children to see the adults in the family being abusive towards one another. They can become worried and anxious, sometimes believing they are the ones at fault. Some will become traumatized and develop PTSD.

## Asylum seekers and young people who have been exposed to war

Asylum seekers usually come from a very different culture to that of the UK. Mental health problems, in particular anxiety, PTSD, and depression, are higher in young people who are refugees or asylum seekers and they are more likely to have somatic presentations of psychological problems. The risk of mental health problems is increased owing to experiences before entering the UK. These include being exposed to war, imprisonment, witnessing or being a victim of sexual or violent abuse, genocide, bereavement, and poverty, as well as having limited access to healthcare.

The process of seeking asylum can also be long, complex, and confusing, particularly for already traumatized young people who have been separated from their primary carers. In addition, the young person can experience prejudice and discrimination. They may also have difficulties communicating, leading them to become isolated.

## Racism

Racism has negative social, economic, and political consequences, as well as direct effects on physical and emotional health. Issues of race and culture can be challenging for the CAMHS clinician. There is a risk of colour or cultural blindness in an atmosphere of political correctness. There may be a fear of causing offence or 'getting it wrong'. However, this ignores the richness involved in difference and diversity. Key issues influencing the client's mental health and recovery are missed and different expressions of illness are ignored. It is a well-documented fact that some cultural groups experience discrimination to a greater degree than others.

Western culture and the 'white race' dominate the social and political system of the UK (Fernando, 1991). The healthcare system, medicines, and the delivery of care make a cultural system. It reflects the symbolic meanings that arise from the social arrangements as well as the clinical institutions where the healthcare is delivered. In any culture, people who are outside the mainstream do not generally have an adequate voice or fair representation. This can affect whether or not young people and their families initially attend and continue to engage in CAMHS, as well as how their needs are recognized and met.

Perceived discrimination has a detrimental effect on mental health. Even if the clinician does not perceive racism to be an issue for the cultural group to which the young person belongs, they still have to consider it in relation to that young person and their family. On the other hand, the clinician ought not presume discrimination is the main or only cause of the young person's distress. The clinician needs to have an open mind to the possibilities for that person, thereby not under- or over-estimating the impact of discrimination.

## Risk to self

Being a risk to oneself can take many forms, including deliberate self-harm, acting in daring and courageous ways even in the face of adversity, substance misuse, putting oneself in a position to be exploited, and neglecting oneself. Young people who are a risk to themselves may benefit from seeing CAMHS, particularly anyone that is deliberately self-harming, has suicidal thoughts or has attempted suicide.

Any young person who has attempted suicide needs to be urgently assessed by CAMHS. What looks like a suicide attempt may not be so and what looks like self-harm may in fact be a suicide attempt. In CAMHS, the terms failed suicide, attempted suicide, parasuicide, deliberate self-harm, and self-mutilation are used to communicate the following:

- *Failed suicide* is where death would have occurred had the person not been found in time or the method had worked.
- *Attempted suicide* is where the person meant to kill themselves but was unsuccessful.
- *Parasuicide* involves an event that resembles a suicide but death was not intended, for example, the young person took an overdose but did not want to kill themselves.

- *Deliberate self-harm* is where the person repeatedly hurts themselves without any intention of causing death.
- *Self-mutilation* involves intentionally changing the shape of the body.

NICE (2004b, 2011, 2013c, 2014) have published a number of documents about deliberate self-harm and suicide. These are also issues addressed in many of the other mental health-related NICE guidelines.

A young person may also be a risk to themselves because of a physical disability, ill-health or a learning disability. Some young people put themselves in situations where they may be at a high risk of exploitation and abuse, such as by joining a gang or running away. A young person who is not attending school is also considered a risk to themselves, as it may not be clear where they are and what they are doing when they should be in class, and they are much less likely to achieve their full potential.

## Deliberate self-harm

Deliberate self-harm (DSH) refers to an act that involves inflicting injuries on one's own body. It is also known as self-injury, cutting, self-abuse, and self-mutilation. DSH is more common than people realize and can take many forms, including cutting that varies from superficial scratches to deep wounds that require stitches. It can also involve rubbing and picking skin to create sores, burning and scalding, hitting and punching oneself, inserting and swallowing objects, pulling out eyelashes and hair, and biting and tearing skin.

DSH also includes running away, staying out late, suicide, sexual promiscuity, acting in daring ways, impulsivity, binge drinking, and experimenting with drugs. Each person's experience of self-harm is different, unique to them. Once the young person can understand what underlies the DSH and how it has functioned for them, they can begin to find new ways of coping. DSH is often mistaken for a suicide attempt but people who self-harm are usually very clear about the difference between the two. It is not about dying, rather about a way of trying to cope and carry on with life. As a result, many people hide their self-harming behaviour, keeping it a secret because of shame, fear, and humiliation.

Self-harming almost always happens in response to painful or difficult events or circumstances. Often no single cause can be identified. DSH is also often related to low self-esteem, alienation, and can be a way of punishing oneself. Some young people find that current situations and events that evoke past distress trigger episodes of hurting themselves. Often these events are reminiscent of past experiences, such as not being heard, feeling rejected or guilty, or feeling unsafe.

DSH can be a way of avoiding feelings. It can numb or distract from distress. For others, it is the only way of avoiding suicide. It can also be a form of communication if one's feelings are being ignored or one is unable to express oneself.

### Suicide

Almost everyone feels sad or lonely at times. Young people can feel like no one really likes them, that they are a failure, they upset everyone, and no one would care if they were dead. They may feel angry but unable to say so, or feel hopeless about the future. These feelings may lead to some young people trying to kill themselves. Several upsetting things may occur over a short time and one more upset or rejection may be the last straw.

In adolescence, suicide is one of the three main causes of death. In young people between the ages of 11 and 15, suicidal thoughts triple in frequency, parallel to the reported rise in attempted and lethal suicides. Young people who attempt suicide are often experiencing very upset feelings or difficult problems for the first time. They don't know how to remedy the situation, become overwhelmed, and see no way out.

There are approximately 13 suicides per 100,000 of 15–19-year-olds in the UK each year. The incidence is higher among male youth, who are less likely to show signs of distress beforehand. About three in five young people who attempt suicide show signs of emotional or behavioural difficulties in the months prior to the attempt without finding help. In adolescence, although boys are three to four times more likely to take their own lives than girls, girls attempt suicide about three times more often.

Approximately 15 per cent of young people who attempt suicide eventually kill themselves at some point in their lives. Suicidal tendencies are not always reflected by sadness, although people recovering from depression are more likely to end their lives. Also, once a suicide plan has been made, the person may feel better and appear calmer and happier.

The decision to attempt suicide is often made quickly without thinking it through. At the time, the young person just wants their problems to disappear, and see no way of seeking help – the only way out is to kill themselves. Such impulsive attempts are very hard to assess.

Anyone under 16 who presents at an emergency department having deliberately self-harmed should be admitted to a paediatric ward, and a CAMHS assessment be conducted. On discharge, the young person should receive a follow-up assessment appointment within 7 working days.

## Risk to others

The risk a young person poses to others comes in many forms, such as violence and aggression, offending behaviours, sexually harmful behaviours, and gang membership. Although not exhaustive, each of these will be addressed in turn from a child and adolescent mental health perspective.

Although forensic CAMHS specializes in assessing and managing the risk of violence and offending behaviour, the risk to others is a matter for all CAMHS to consider.

## Violence and aggression

The Structured Assessment for Violence Risk in Youth (SAVRY) (Borum et al., 2006) is a tool used by CAMHS to assess risk and plan interventions in relation to the risk of violence in 12–18-year-olds. It offers a 24-item, systematic and empirically grounded framework for considering risk.

Violence is an intentional act of physical battery that causes injury to another person (although this could be sexual, sexual violence is considered separately). Threatening someone with a weapon is also considered a violent act. The areas of risk explored here are considered in more detail in the SAVRY manual.

There are two types of aggression – reactive and proactive. *Reactive aggression* is a retaliatory response to perceived provocation and is normally accompanied by feelings of anger and impulsive behaviour. *Proactive aggression*, in contrast, is usually unprovoked and has an intended outcome. It is not impulsive and tends not to be accompanied by angry feelings. Anger management problems are associated with a high risk of reactive aggression, while low empathy and lack of remorse and callous and unemotional traits are associated with proactive aggression.

Historical risk factors are based on past experience or behaviours. CAMHS needs to get as much information as possible from a variety of sources to corroborate the facts. Young people can over- or underplay their involvement in violent and aggressive acts in response to who they are talking to and what image they want to portray. And the best predictor of future violence is prior violence. The age of onset of violent or aggressive behaviour, its severity and frequency, and when the last act was committed, all can increase the risk profile. Research has found that non-violent offending behaviour, suicide attempts, and deliberate self-harm also reflect a higher risk of violence, which may indicate other factors are at play, such as poor coping mechanisms or stress.

In general, having a supportive family, community, and peer environment will contribute towards a young person's resilience (Olsson et al., 2003), so friendships, social support, strong attachments and bonds are important. It is through the experience of groups and a gradual understanding of acceptable group behaviour that young people learn that immediate gratification is not always possible.

The family group potentially offers a safe group experience where children and young people learn about boundaries, delayed gratification, frustrated plans, and conflict management. The young person's experience of being parented or cared for is also important, as poor parental management, parental criminality, the witnessing of domestic abuse, being abused or neglected, and early disruptions to care are all associated with an increase in the risk profile for a young person.

The peer group experience offers an important means of teaching a young person. Groups of friends are generally seen as a protective factor, especially if there is a network of prosocial peers or a prosocial adult with whom the young person has a relationship. Although this appears a logical conclusion, it presumes that groups are always a positive influence. Young people are social beings and although in general social relationships are positive and protective, some groups can be a negative influence, and peer delinquency has been shown to be a significant risk factor. Violence can be both tolerated by the group and used to exert a cohesive, unifying effect through shared risks, loyalty, and secrecy. Likewise, peer rejection and not being liked by any or many peers can leave a young person vulnerable to violence. In some circumstances, what is considered maladaptive behaviour can be a natural response to abusive, violent relationships and group dynamics.

Young people who have been deprived of healthy group or family experiences are less likely to have had positive developmental experiences. They may be less able to tolerate deferred gratification and may engage in behaviour that facilitates immediate gratification and increased risk. Both families and peer groups may not be able to provide a healthy and helpful developmental experience in a safe way, which can be exacerbated by community disorganization, another risk factor for violence.

Young people who live in areas where there is offending behaviour and possibly gang activity are unavoidably exposed to risks such as anti-social behaviour, crime, poverty, stigmatization, and fear. Within the school context, factors that increase the risk of violence include poor attendance, low interest and commitment, and poor achievement. Similarly, not complying with other statutory services, such as youth offending services and the associated court orders, also increases risk. These young people often come across as having negative cognitions and attitudes towards authority, crime and life, and these are associated with a higher level of risk. These may be observed as perceived hostility, fear of victimization, and lack of perceived opportunities to achieve.

Impulsivity, risk-taking, and substance misuse are also associated with a higher risk profile. In addition, mental health problems, such as depression, anxiety, and attention deficit hyperactivity disorder (ADHD) have an impact on the resilience of a young person.

### Offending behaviours

Young people may be involved in offending behaviour, whether or not they have a conviction or have had a caution. These young people are at a higher risk of experiencing mental health difficulties. Offending behaviour covers different types of behaviour and can be committed as a group or alone. Types of offending behaviour include anti-social behaviour, car crime, dishonesty, drugs offences, hate crime, sexual offences, and violent crime.

**Sexually harmful behaviours**

In relation to the risk of sexually harmful behaviour, tools similar to the SAVRY have been developed. The Estimated Risk of Adolescent Sexual Offence Recidivism (ERASOR; Worling and Curwen, 2001) is complemented by the Desistence for Adolescents who Sexually Harm (DASH-13; Worling, 2013), which is used to understand the protective factors. These have been designed for use with 12–18-year-olds who have committed an offence of a sexual nature, whether or not they have been convicted. It is important to note that although most research has been in relation to males who engage in sexually harmful behaviour, females also commit sexual offences.

Sexually harmful behaviour towards others involves not just penetrative or non-penetrative sexual acts but also distributing or making sexual images. Young people with learning or social communication difficulties may display sexually harmful behaviour.

When assessing the risk of committing a sexual offence, various factors need to be considered. The ERASOR lists these as:

1. Sexual interests, attitudes, and behaviours
2. Historical sexual assaults
3. Psychosocial functioning
4. Family and environmental functioning
5. Treatment.

ERASOR goes on to detail the current evidence and aids the experienced CAMHS clinician can use to assess the level of risk of future sexually harmful behaviour. In summary, young people who have a deviant sexual interest or who become aroused sexually by young children or violent assaults, are preoccupied with sexual thoughts, have a supportive attitude to sexually harmful behaviour, and are unwillingness to change are at a higher risk of future sexually harmful behaviour.

The section of ERASOR on sexually harmful behaviour explores the nature and frequency of previous assaults as well as the number and type of victims. The following two sections of the instrument detail the social groups and attitudes of the young person and their immediate family and community environment. The final section of ERASOR details the previous interventions that have been tried, the young person's engagement with them, and opportunities for future treatment.

The DASH-13 is a helpful checklist of factors that a clinician can use to determine what the young person displays in terms of resilience. These include prosocial sexual arousal, prosocial sexual attitudes, hope for a healthy sexual future, successful completion of sexual offence-specific treatment, awareness of consequences of sexual reoffending, and environmental controls that match risk to reoffend sexually; the other seven factors address prosocial functioning.

### Gang membership

Gang membership and affiliation are increasingly considered within the context of a CAMHS risk assessment. In the UK, gangs tend not to be formal organizations and the term 'membership' could be misleading (Aldridge and Medina, 2008). For ease of reference, the Eurogang definition of a gang is adopted here: 'any durable, street-orientated youth group whose involvement in illegal activity is part of its group identity' (Esbensen and Weerman, 2005). The key terms within this definition are (Weerman et al., 2009: 148):

- *Durability* means the gang has existed several months or more and refers to the group that continues despite the turnover of its members.
- *Street-orientated* means the group spends a lot of group time outside home, work, and school, and often on streets, in malls, in parks, in cars, and so on.
- *Youth* means that members' *average* age is in the teens or early twenties.
- *Illegal activity* generally means delinquent or criminal behavior, not just bothersome activity.
- *Identity* refers to the group's, not individual members', self-image.

The literature suggests that gang membership has a detrimental effect on a young person's mental health. CAMHS is often a member of a strategic group considering how to tackle the 'gang problem' in a locality.

Gang membership may be associated with higher rates of ADHD, PTSD, and callous and unemotional traits. These and the status conferred on the young person by group membership lead to more risk-taking behaviour and a lack of regard for the consequences of their actions, often leading to more serious and violent offences being committed.

## Risk management

Risk management is a key role within CAMHS. It involves developing strategies to prevent potential adverse events from occurring, or minimizing the harm or distress caused by them. The risks are never going to be eliminated completely and CAMHS will work with the young person and their family to weigh up the potential benefits against the harms of choosing one action over another.

What do you think are effective risk management strategies?

CAMHS uses a range of risk management strategies. It is good practice to develop the risk management plan with the young person and their family. The principles set out in Chapter 11 in relation to developing a care plan are relevant to the process of developing a risk management plan.

Help the young person to:

- Be involved.
- Be creative – what is important to the young person, what do they respond well to?
- Be flexible by coaching them to come up with ideas.
- Own the plan and its implementation.
- Involve the family.
- Involve other people who are in the young person's life: teachers, family friends.
- Think about where and when the risks are higher.
- Think about what makes them feel and stay safe: people, places, activities – for each person this might be different.
- Be honest about what is working and what is not working.

When a risk management plan has been developed, it is essential that it be communicated to all relevant parties. This will mean that the clinician will have to negotiate with the young person to balance the risk against the young person's right to confidentiality. Ideally, the risk management plan should involve the roles and responsibilities of each family member and professional that is known to the young person. The plan should also include emergency contact details and contingency plans for when things go wrong. Each plan is individualized but will contain some common features, such as emergency phone numbers, details of the local duty system and local support services. The more individualized parts of the risk management plan will be actions that the young person and their family find helpful when managing their symptoms.

Each locality will have a process for managing emergencies outside of the standard CAMHS working hours. This may be supported by a protocol, developed with partner agencies, that covers what happens in an emergency. During CAMHS working hours, most localities have a duty system where a clinician, manager, and consultant psychiatrist are available to manage any emergencies that arise, whether the young person is currently known to the service or a new referral to CAMHS. Most local CAMHS will have established working relationships and protocols with the emergency department so that young people who present there have swift access to a mental health assessment.

Some teams use standardized paper forms or electronic versions to document a risk assessment. As it should be copied to the young person and their family, it is important that it is written in a language the young person can understand. The CAMHS clinician needs to be mindful that a young person may not want to end their appointment with a printed version of the risk management plan out of fear of someone else seeing it. They may prefer that the family be entrusted with it or that it be sent by text or email in a format that makes sense to them. It is important that their confidentiality is not compromised and that they have the information for emergencies readily available.

A risk management plan should be reviewed on an ongoing basis. The clinician might set a review date with the young person and their family, but will review it sooner if the risk profile changes or it is found that the strategies are not working for that individual.

Imagine someone approached you and said they wanted to write a risk management plan in order to keep you safe.

- What sort of things would run through your mind?
- How would you like the person to approach the subject?
- What questions come to mind?
- How would you like it to look? What format would you prefer?

## Learning lessons

No matter how robust a risk assessment and a risk management plan might be, risk cannot be eliminated. Unfortunately, terrible things happen to, are witnessed by, or are done by children and young people. CAMHS owes it to all the young people and families involved that they learn from things that go wrong.

A serious care review might be undertaken locally when a serious incident occurs that involves all the agencies having contact with the child and family. This is usually when a child dies (including suicide), when abuse or neglect is known or suspected to be a factor, when a child sustains a potentially life-threatening injury, or where the health and development of the child have been seriously and permanently impaired. A review will also be conducted when a child has been seriously sexually abused, or if the case raises concerns about inter-agency working that is meant to protect the child.

Serious case reviews are not enquiries into how a child has died or who is culpable; this is the role of the coroner and criminal courts. Instead, they are used to establish if there are lessons to be learned about how professionals and agencies work together to safeguard children. They aim to identify the lessons and how agencies will act on them. There is an expectation that all agencies will change as a result and there will be tangible improvements in inter-agency working to better safeguard children.

An independent investigation into adverse events in mental health services is conducted when a person who is or has been under the care of specialist mental health services in the previous six months commits a homicide. Such an investigation will also be conducted when it is necessary to comply with the State's obligations under Article 2 of the European Convention on Human Rights. That is where the State is, or may be, responsible for a death. An independent investigation may also be called if there was a significant systemic service failure.

When someone dies as result of domestic violence, the law requires that all the professionals involved in the case must conduct a multi-agency review of what happened so that they can identify what needs to be changed to reduce the risk of it happening again. Other investigations that might be conducted include an internal serious untoward incident investigation, an independent investigation, and a domestic homicide review. Each health organization will have a policy and protocols in place for how they investigate serious untoward incidents, including multi-agency and independent reviews. These will result in recommendations and an action plan to improve services and learn lessons.

This chapter has looked at the complex area of risk, risk assessment, and risk management in CAMHS. This included clinical risks such as safeguarding children and adults and the risk young people pose to themselves and others. The chapter concluded with risk management and the need for lessons to be learned from serious incidents.

## Key messages

- Risk assessment and risk management are important within CAMHS and cover multiple domains.
- Children and young people can be a risk to themselves or a risk to others, or they can be at risk from others or the environment.
- Risk management is most effective when it involves the young person.
- Communication is key to good risk management.

## Further reading

Geldard, K. (2009) *Practical Interventions for Young People at Risk*. London: Sage.
Powell, C. (2011) *Safeguarding and Child Protection for Nurses, Midwives and Health Visitors: A Practical Guide*. Maidenhead: Open University Press.

# 11 Interventions

In this chapter, a range of interventions will be introduced, starting with the basics. More specific interventions will then be covered in sections on parenting, consultation, care planning, education, therapies, and psychopharmacology. Next, compulsory interventions are considered before a final section on transitioning a young person to adult services.

The interventions provided by CAMHS are many and varied. Previously, CAMHS had been asked to report on performance indicators and to follow evidence-based practice for discrete illnesses, as defined by diagnostic criteria, rather than referring to the quality of person-centred, holistic care. This is not the relational language of caring, but the language of the market. Recently, there has been a shift, not away from performance indicators and evidence-based practice, but a move to include the elements of care, service user satisfaction, and outcomes.

The evidence CAMHS bases its treatment interventions on is the best available evidence at the present time, and will change and develop over time. Interventions are not the specific remit of a single professional discipline, and with the appropriate training and support, CAMHS clinicians are able to provide a wide range of treatments.

## Getting the basics right

There are some basic requirements to maintaining good physical and mental health. When not attended to, there may be a negative impact on the mental health of children and young people. Occasionally, the cause of the difficulty, such as a behavioural or emotional problem, can be resolved if some of these basic requirements for a healthy life are addressed. The basic requirements for good mental health include physical healthcare needs, sleep, diet, and exercise, each of which will be covered in turn. Alongside this, good mental health promotion is essential for both the prevention and treatment of difficulties.

### Physical health

Traditionally, CAMHS has focused on mental health not physical health, leaving that to GPs, health visitors, and school nurses. The exceptions to this are when the young person is an in-patient or when they have had a mental health problem and the risk to physical health is very high, such as an eating disorder.

Achieving 'parity of esteem' for people with mental health problems, whereby mental health is valued as highly as physical health, is high on the agenda nationally. This mandate has often been used to ensure mental health services are given as high a profile as physical healthcare. Those with mental health problems are known to have worse outcomes in terms of physical health. Parity of esteem also means that those with mental health problems also have their physical healthcare needs attended to.

Physical healthcare is an important consideration when working with a child or young person with mental health problems, as the physical problem could be causing the mental health problem, be associated with it or even exacerbating it. The CAMHS clinician will have covered physical health needs and difficulties, including dental care, pain and chronic conditions, in the initial assessment. Any issues that come to light during the assessment may form part of the recommendations for improving the health of the young person in question.

Many CAMHS will weigh and measure a young person at their initial assessment. They will then repeat these measures at regular intervals, or more frequently if required. Subtle and unexplained changes may be the first indication that the young person's appetite has changed, as a consequence of mood or the side-effects of medication.

## Sleep

Children and young people need long periods of uninterrupted sleep for optimal growth and development. Any sleep problems can create or exacerbate mental health problems. A vicious cycle can be created whereby a lack of sleep exacerbates a mental health problem, resulting in further difficulty sleeping. Sleep deprivation has a negative effect on mood, increases aggression and anger, and impacts control of one's impulses.

Both going to sleep and staying asleep can be a problem, and struggles between young people and their parents with regard to sleep can cause tension and have a negative effect on family relationships. The case of a young child will need to be managed differently from that of an adolescent. Parents of younger children need to learn about the importance of sleep and the positive impact a good night's sleep can have on a child's behaviour. The parents will need to commit to a consistent and committed approach to how they manage bedtimes and night-time waking. Without this commitment, a positive outcome will be less likely and frustrations within the family can grow.

For adolescents, it is important that they take ownership of their sleep routine, otherwise there is a risk of them rebelling against any suggestions. The clinician can suggest ways to help a young person establish good sleep hygiene. The young person should exercise during the day but not just before bedtime. They can be encouraged to go to bed at the same time each night, adopt a relaxing night-time routine, and get up at the same time in the morning. Caffeine and foods and drinks high in sugar should be avoided. In the event that the young person cannot sleep, they should get up and do something relaxing, such as listening to music or reading until they feel sleepy.

Televisions and mobile phones are an unavoidable part of life and it may be unrealistic to remove these from the bedroom, particularly if the young person uses their phone as an alarm. Discussing this with a young person could result in a compromise, such as leaving the phone, with the alarm on, on the other side of the bedroom, thus removing the temptation to play games and message friends during the night.

## Diet

Diet is not just important when working with young people who have an eating disorder – it is important for all young people. The food a young person eats can affect their mood, their behaviour, and the way their brain functions. And being hungry can make people irritable and restless. Research suggests some nutrients can impact mood, sleep patterns, energy levels, and thinking. When children miss breakfast, it is associated with reductions in fluency, motivation, and problem-solving ability.

Although it has been suggested that foods high in sugar cause hyperactivity in children, research does not support this. However, it does support the association between a diet high in sugar and poor dental health, which can cause chronic pain and in turn behavioural problems. Some research suggests that fish oils may help with symptoms of hyperactivity.

## Exercise

Exercise is known to have many benefits for maintaining and improving mental health. When exercising, endorphins are released into the brain, which makes people feel happier. Exercise also aids sleep and concentration and helps maintain a healthy weight, bones and muscles. There are secondary gains also, in that exercise promotes socialization and a sense of belonging when participating in team sports.

## Mental health promotion

Improving the mental health literacy of the young person and their family is an important component of the treatment plan. Poor mental health literacy raises ethical questions because it is a barrier to healthcare and results in poor health outcomes. This part of the treatment plan, also known as psycho-education, could involve the clinician directly educating the young person and their family. Alternatively, they could be directed to helpful websites, books, support groups or DVDs. It is more likely that a clinician will use a combination of these methods and for the young person, family, and clinician to come together again to discuss what has been learnt and address any questions.

Many interventions also involve working with parents and supporting them as they improve their own parenting skills, and so we will consider these next.

## Parenting

The internal and external problems and strengths families possess are many and varied. They can manifest in any or every part of the family, including the parents and the children. Also, what is considered the primary problem may not be a stand-alone issue. Many factors will likely contribute to the situation the young person and their family find themselves in. In addition, there is the question of whether the family want help, are able to access help or know what help is available. This in itself can be a problem.

Although the young person is at the centre of any CAMHS assessment and ongoing work, many factors – including other people, organizations, the environment, and the government – will exert an influence to some extent. Parents or other primary caregivers will usually be closest to the child or young person and so have a significant impact on them.

How a child experiences parenting is an important part of how they develop, and every child needs a foundation of love and care. Being a good parent means different things to different people and is strongly influenced by experience and culture. Fundamentally good parenting provides a warm, secure home life with rules and boundaries where the child is able to develop self-esteem and respect for others.

When a young person has a mental health problem, their parents may have been told for years that their child is behaving badly and that they are bad parents. They may feel they are to blame and that the root of the problem is their parenting style. This is rarely the case but parenting support and training can be an effective part of any treatment plan. This may appear somewhat contradictory to parents, as on the one hand they are told their parenting is not to blame but on the other are offered parent training. CAMHS needs to handle the situation with sensitivity, explaining that parenting a child or young person with a mental health problem can be challenging, and that different techniques can be employed. Support groups, where the parents of children with similar mental health problems come together, are often helpful.

Parenting support and education in CAMHS can take the form of individual sessions with a clinician or group programmes. Many formal parenting programmes are evidence-based and delivered by CAMHS, either alone or in partnership with other agencies. These include Triple P, the Incredible Years Programme, and the Strengthening Families Programme. To ensure these programmes are highly accessible, the time at which they are delivered, childcare arrangements, and the venue for any programme must be taken into consideration. Some areas offer a parallel programme for young people, with a mechanism for parents and young people to come together.

Another type of intervention is consultation, which we look at next.

## Consultation

Consultation with those involved in the care of children and young people is an important part of the service CAMHS offers. Consultation can aid early intervention and ensure referrals are appropriate, made in a timely manner, and accompanied by the relevant information. Consultation can be in relation to an individual or group of children, who are or are not known to CAMHS. Any consultation needs to have been discussed with the family if identifying information is to be disclosed; if not, the information must be anonymized.

A consultation with CAMHS can be used to think through any concerns in relation to a young person's mental health problems. A consultation can clarify the thresholds for a CAMHS service and open up the option of joint working between services. At the beginning of any consultation, the CAMHS practitioner will highlight issues regarding confidentiality, safeguarding, and sharing of information. The parties involved should agree how the consultation will be documented and who will own the information recorded, if this is not already set out in a local protocol. It can be helpful to ask the person seeking the consultation what they hope to achieve and what questions they would like answered by the end of the consultation. At the end of the consultation, there should be a formulation of the difficulties and a plan for moving forward, with or without CAMHS.

Any intervention will be part of a care plan by CAMHS, so the next section considers the importance of good care planning.

## Care planning

To manage any problem brought to their attention, CAMHS will work with the young person and their family to set clear goals and decide any treatments and interventions. Through a process of collaboration, these then form the care plan. By deciding any actions and goals in collaboration with the clinician, the young person and their family will become immediately engaged in the process. To begin, the clinician will identify the general aims and direction the family want to go in. They will then work with the family to develop these into goals. Increasingly in CAMHS these goals are aimed at recovery.

It is important the young person and their family understand the perspective of the clinician because at times the clinician will challenge their views and ideas while simultaneously working in partnership with them. Any challenges should be made specific, and framed in a positive and constructive way. An effective challenge will open the way for the family to think about their situation in new and alternative ways. Although they may not be comfortable with a new way of thinking, it will become clear to them that there are alternatives. It is unlikely that any family will engage with a care plan if they do not feel it meets their needs as they perceive them or they do not understand the plan's rationale.

A care plan needs to recognize that each young person is a unique individual whose best interests must be served. The clinician must never use a template or one-size-fits-all approach. The plan should be developed in accordance with the young person's age and understanding. By doing so, the young person becomes an informed participant. It is important that the care plan is developed in a way that is culturally sensitive and considers the physical, psychological, social, and spiritual needs of the young person and their family in a non-judgemental, non-discriminatory way.

To be effective, the goals and actions in the care plan need to be:

- Specific
- Measurable
- Achievable
- Realistic
- Time-orientated
- Explicit
- Negotiated.

The young person and their family will decide with the clinician what is achievable in a given period of time and how things would look if successful. By doing this, the goals can be expressed as an outcome or a target in a very positive way. The care plan may involve input from other agencies involved in the care of the young person, but the expectation of partners must be realistic and always negotiated with them. An action by a specific person must never be written into a care plan without the person agreeing to its inclusion.

Involving young people and their families in the process of care planning facilitates creative approaches to and presentation of the care plan. In CAMHS, a care plan is usually a written account, either contained within a letter or as a separate document detailing what interventions have been planned. They can be adapted to the developmental needs of the child, for example, using pictures as well as words.

To ensure the goals are not overwhelming, only two or three ought to be developed at any one time. This will increase the likelihood of the young person and their family acting in accordance with the plan and contributing to its success. If a number of goals are identified, they can be prioritized and worked on in order. At review, any remaining goals can be reprioritized if something has had an effect on the outstanding issues.

It can be helpful to think about what the family envisages the situation will look like if the care plan is successful and then revisit it when the care plan is evaluated. At review, the young person and their family can update the clinician on any progress and celebrate any success. The clinician will discuss with them what worked and what did not work, and suggest new approaches to achieving any outstanding goals.

## Interventions in an education setting

Children and young people with mental health problems spend a lot of time at school, and education staff have to manage and teach them within the context of the wider needs of the class. The interface between CAMHS and education usually begins with the referral or assessment. A classroom and playground observation of the child by a CAMHS clinician can offer valuable insight into the young person's difficulties, and is also a time for getting to know the key educational staff in the young person's life and who might contribute to the assessment and treatment plan.

The individual needs of the child need to be balanced with those of their peers. An effective care plan can be developed between CAMHS and the educational setting if it is developed with the young person, their family, and professionals from the two agencies. A care plan is less likely to be effective if CAMHS tries to direct the school staff to respond in a specific way, as the CAMHS worker will not be familiar with the school and classroom context. The education and CAMHS specialists need to work together, sharing their perspectives and expertise.

If medications are to be taken during the school day, it is important for CAMHS to ensure the educational staff are aware of the effects and side-effects of those medications, together with details of when and how much of any medication should be taken. Some medications may make the child or young person very thirsty and, coupled with manic symptoms or impulsivity, they may frequently ask for a drink and then to go to the toilet. Understanding this and allowing them greater access to drinking water and the toilet will help minimize disruption to the rest of the class while helping the young person to manage the side-effects.

Some young people with mental health problems may need additional support in the classroom, a reduced amount of homework or a period of no homework. An agreed means of communication between the teacher, the parent, and CAMHS, such as emails, can greatly assist in the treatment of these young people. Such communication can warn the teacher of particular difficulties that day, the teacher can report back or ensure the parent knows what is happening. CAMHS can monitor progress and ensure early intervention if matters start to deteriorate.

A school can have a designated 'safe place' where the young person can take time out. The school can also designate a staff member whom the young person trusts and to whom they can go if needed.

While an in-patient, a young person may have been a pupil in the hospital school. The specialist teachers in these schools can plan a gradual return to mainstream education and assist the teachers to put in place an individualized plan. Similarly, when a young person has been away from school for a period of time owing to illness, CAMHS can usefully negotiate a graduated return to school, which may include later starting times.

Exams can be particularly stressful times for young people who have mental health problems. The school can be encouraged to put in place extended times, breaks, and other approved supports during examinations.

Next we consider the therapies used in CAMHS as a form of intervention.

## Therapies

The therapies used in CAMHS have different philosophical backgrounds. Some are very structured whereas others are completely left to develop as the sessions evolve. Therapy can be delivered individually, as a family, or in a general group setting. Whatever the setting, the therapist will need to be appropriately trained and supervised. The therapies described here are those most frequently used in a CAMHS setting.

### Behaviour therapy

Behaviour therapy is based on the theory of classical conditioning and the idea that all behaviour is learned. This form of therapy aims to support the young person to learn more adaptive behaviours. It focuses on the present and does not attempt to address the causes. Some techniques that may be used are systematic desensitization, aversion therapy, and flooding. It is rare in CAMHS for behaviour therapy to be used alone.

### Child psychoanalytic psychotherapy

Child psychoanalytic psychotherapy is also known as child psychodynamic psychotherapy. It draws on theories and practices of analytical psychology and psychoanalysis and helps the young person to understand and resolve their problems. The therapist carefully observes the child or young person and responds to what they might be communicating through their behaviour and play. This form of therapy aims to achieve deep-seated change in personality and emotional development.

### Cognitive behavioural therapy

Cognitive behavioural therapists work with how a young person thinks and what they do. The young person can meet one-to-one with the therapist, attend groups or do CBT online. The young person will learn about their thoughts, feelings, actions, and physical reactions. The therapist will devise 'experiments' for the young person to test out their assumptions and thoughts about a situation. This may involve homework to be undertaken with the family. Psycho-education is a key element in this form of therapy.

## Dialectical behaviour therapy

Dialectical behaviour therapy (DBT) was developed from CBT and is used with young people who have difficulties regulating their emotions. It works on the premise that the present circumstances do not determine the future; they are merely the starting point. Treatment emphasizes the psychosocial aspects of the difficulties the young person is experiencing. DBT is a supportive and collaborative approach and particularly good results have been achieved with young people who deliberately self-harm or act impulsively (James et al., 2008). Treatment usually involves both group and individual sessions and work centres around emotional regulation, mindfulness, interpersonal effectiveness, and distress tolerance.

## Family Partnership Model

The Family Partnership Model (FPM) enables CAMHS clinicians to develop effective partnerships with parents and use a structured and flexible relational, goal-orientated approach to achieve the best possible outcome. FPM explicitly builds on and uses family strengths and expertise, specifies the practitioner's qualities and skills, and focuses on the helping tasks that enable parents and families to change and achieve the very best for their children and themselves.

## Occupational therapy

Occupational therapy is based on the concept that occupation is essential if people are to have good health and well-being. Occupational therapists assess the underlying difficulties that impair the young person's ability to manage and interact with everyday tasks.

Occupational therapy plays an important role within the CAMHS in-patient setting but also has a role, although is less commonly found, in community CAMHS. Occupational therapy can provide treatment for motor coordination difficulties, which are sometimes identified in young people diagnosed with ADHD. The benefits of occupational therapy can also be applied to neuro-development services.

In the CAMHS in-patient setting, occupational therapy forms one of the core aspects of the treatment plan for the young person. For young people with eating disorders, management of their physical activity will be important.

### Speech and language therapy

Speech and language therapy has long been used when working with young people with social communication difficulties. More recently, it has been introduced to the youth justice system with promising results. Speech and language therapists play an important role in identifying unmet speech and communication needs. The interventions used in this form of therapy can help prevent and reduce re-offending by increasing verbal communication skills. It enables young people to engage better in any programmes aimed at preventing them from re-offending.

### Interpersonal therapy

Interpersonal therapy (IPT), which has been adapted for work with adolescents (IPT-A), is a form of therapy where the young person works with a suitably trained therapist on a one-to-one basis for a time-limited period. This structured therapy attempts to replace conflictual and unfulfilling relationships with ones that are less conflictual and more meaningful. The sessions focus on conflict with other people, life changes that affect how the young person feels, grief and loss, and starting and maintaining relationships.

### Play therapy

Play therapy uses play rather than words as a form of communication. The aim is to assist the child to modify their behaviour and build healthy relationships, and help them to find healthier ways of communicating, develop relationships, and increase resiliency.

### Systemic family psychotherapy

In CAMHS, systemic family psychotherapy is sometimes referred to as systemic therapy or family therapy. It focuses on relationships and sees the importance of context in understanding and in shaping behaviours. Systemic therapy challenges the idea that there are simple, straightforward causes of problems; instead, it looks at the system, which it sees as the sum of its parts.

Systemic therapy works with narrative ideas and places an emphasis on change. There are many different approaches and models but most family therapists in CAMHS use an integrative approach to fit the therapy with the family and their presenting difficulties. There is a focus on change rather than finding the 'cause' of the problem in this form of therapy. The therapist works with strengths and the system rather than the individual.

### Mentalization-based therapies

Mentalization is the ability to think about thinking. The goal of mentalization-based therapies is to help the young person to recognize and understand their own emotional and mental state as well as that of other people and how this affects behaviour. They learn to 'step back' from their thoughts about themselves and others and examine them to determine whether they are valid.

### Mindfulness

Mindfulness is about experiencing life in the here and now rather than going along with automatic and unhelpful ways of thinking. Mindfulness is a technique that takes time to develop and requires some effort. Meditation is one way of teaching mindfulness. Its aim is to allow the person to consider the whole experience, excluding nothing. It is a non-judgemental approach that takes one experience at a time. Becoming more aware of the present moment can help young people to enjoy the world around them and to understand themselves better by taking time and using sight, sound, smell, and taste.

### E-therapies

Social media, the internet, and information technology are an integral part of the life of young people, thus it would make sense to consider them in any assessment and intervention. Some have gone beyond considering the information technology the young person uses and have developed assessment and treatment programmes that are available and administered electronically.

In 2014, the National Collaborating Centre for Mental Health published 'E-therapies Systematic Review for Children and Young People with Mental Health Problems'. This is a comprehensive review of the use of information technology in the treatment of children and young people with mental health problems.

Computerized therapy programmes are in the early stage of development but there is evidence to suggest that they may be helpful when used alongside mental health service input. They need to be offered free of charge and support the promotion of the young person's autonomy over their treatment. Currently, computerized CBT for depression has the most evidence to support its efficacy.

## Psychopharmacology

There is an extensive and rapidly developing evidence base for prescribing medications to children and young people with mental health problems. The study of using medications to address the mood, sensation, thinking, and behaviour of people is called psychopharmacology and the medications used are sometimes called psychotropic drugs. General issues relating to psychopharmacological interventions as specific disorders are covered in Chapters 8 and 9.

Medications can be an effective part of treatment for child and adolescent mental health problems but this may raise concerns and questions for the young person and their families. Furthermore, professionals from partner agencies and friends and family may have their own views of medication use based on strongly held ethical or religious beliefs or a misunderstanding of the evidence base. There are some understandable concerns and controversies regarding the prescription of psychotropic medications for children and young people. These need to be kept in mind while retaining a balanced view of the utility of psychopharmacology. There have been few randomized controlled trials with children, meaning most of these medications are not licensed for use with children. Because of this, there is a limited evidence base and this needs to be weighed against the risks to the young person if not prescribed medication.

CAMHS will explain in full the reasons for prescribing any medication, what benefits the medication should provide, as well as possible risks, adverse effects, and alternative treatments. Psychiatric medications should not be used as the sole form of treatment. CAMHS practitioners will also understand the complex and challenging issues that might warrant prescribing different medications, whether singly or in combination, at different times during the course of a young person's treatment.

Although all CAMHS practitioners with possess knowledge and skills in relation to child and adolescent psychopharmacology, all medications are prescribed by a psychiatrist or non-medical prescriber, such as a nurse. All non-medical prescribers will have undertaken specialist training and passed exams. All CAMHS practitioners will know the risks and benefits of prescribing any medication to a young person. They will also know when to refer to an appropriate professional for further assessment and, where appropriate, prescribing.

Before commencing medication, the young person will have had a thorough mental health assessment. In some cases, the assessment will include a full CAMHS assessment, as detailed in Chapter 4, but may also include a physical examination, laboratory tests such as blood tests, and other procedures such as an electrocardiogram (ECG) or electroencephalogram (EEG).

Prescribing regimes will vary and with developments in pharmaceuticals, new drugs may become an option. Any co-morbidity and the complexity and individuality of the young person's presentation will be considered. Although not an exhaustive list, psychopharmacological interventions can be used with obsessive-compulsive disorder (OCD), tics and Tourette's syndrome, anxiety disorder, pervasive development disorder (PDD) and autism spectrum disorder (ASD), early-onset psychosis, depression and learning disabilities, bedwetting, eating disorders, severe aggression, and sleep problems.

We now address compulsory detention or treatment, which will be followed by a brief section about the transition of a young person to adult mental health services (AMHS).

# Compulsory detention and treatment

Children and young people can be detained and treated against their will in certain circumstances. Occasionally, the common law will be used if there is a life-threatening situation and no one is able to provide consent. In other circumstances, the Mental Health Act 2007 is used. There are also circumstances under the Children Act 1989 and the Crime and Disorder Act 1998 where a young person can be detained or treated.

### Mental Health Act

The Mental Health Act 1983 was amended in 2007 and is the legal framework that allows treatment for mental disorders. The Mental Health Act 2007 can be used with children and young people because there is no lower age limit. It will be determined whether a young person is able to decide for themselves about their assessment and treatment. It is important to confirm the validity of any consent provided.

The Mental Health Act is applied in the same way for 16- and 17-year-olds as it is with adults who have the capacity to consent or refuse informal admission. For young people below the age of 16 who are not Gillick-competent (as described in Chapter 6), the person who has parental responsibility can consent to their admission and treatment.

Those who lack capacity to consent to admission can be admitted under the Mental Capacity Act 2005. This must not amount to a detention, which would be subject to the Deprivation of Liberty Safeguards (DOLS). These safeguards are part of the Mental Capacity Act 2005 and aim to make sure that people in care homes, hospitals, and supported accommodation are looked after in a way that does not inappropriately restrict their freedom.

If a young person is detained under the Mental Health Act (sectioned), they must remain in hospital for either an assessment or treatment until they are well enough to be discharged. The young person will have had to have been very ill and required help urgently. This usually means the young person was a risk to themselves or other people.

Young people who are sectioned under the Mental Health Act have rights, just as adults do. The young person's nearest relative must be consulted and they can object to the child being sectioned; if their objection is considered reasonable, a Section 3 can be prevented (see Box 11.1 for an explanation of the sections under the Mental Health Act). The young person also has the right to an independent advocate and to appeal against any section to the Mental Health Tribunal. Treatment can be given without consent for up to three months if the care team believe it essential.

The young person can speak to the Care Quality Commission (CQC) about any aspect of their care and treatment. After discharge, the young person will be entitled to aftercare under Section 117. All detained young people should have their rights read to them and given to them in an accessible and developmentally appropriate format.

---

### Box 11.1: Types of section

Different sections can be used under different circumstances and for different reasons. In summary:

- *Section 2* is an assessment order that lasts up to 28 days.
- *Section 3* is a treatment order that initially lasts up to 6 months but can be renewed for a further 6 months. After this, the order lasts for up to one year.
- *Section 4* is an emergency order that lasts up to 72 hours.
- *Section 5(2)* is a doctor's holding power. It can only be used to detain in hospital a person who has consented to admission on an informal basis but then changed their mind and wishes to leave.
- *Section 5(4)* is a nurse's holding power. It can be applied to the same group of patients as those that may be detained under Section 5(2) as outlined above. It lasts up to 6 hours.
- *Section 135* is a magistrates' order. It gives police officers the right to enter the property and to take the person to a 'place of safety', which is usually either a police station or a mental health hospital ward.
- *Section 136* allows a police officer to take a person whom they consider to be mentally disordered to a 'place of safety'.
- *Section 35* and *Section 36* are similar to Section 2 and Section 3 respectively, but are used for people awaiting trial for a serious crime. It provides an alternative to remanding a mentally disordered person in prison.
- *Section 37* is a treatment order. It is applied to people convicted of a serious crime that is punishable by imprisonment. It provides an alternative to a mentally disordered person being punished by imprisonment.
- *Section 41* is imposed by the Crown Court. It is universally imposed without limit of time.

---

### Children Act

The Children Act 1989 can also restrict the liberty of a young person. A secure accommodation order under Section 25 of the Children Act 1989 allows a person under 18 to be kept in secure accommodation with the purpose of restricting their liberty if they have a history of absconding from other placements and they are likely to cause significant harm to themselves or injure others. This Act allows for court involvement in individual treatment decisions but it does not specifically address mental disorders.

### Crime and Disorder Act

Under the Crime and Disorder Act 1998, young people who are convicted of an offence may be subject to a youth rehabilitation order (YRO). This YRO can have mental health treatment requirements. Although not compulsory, non-compliance can have serious consequences for the young person, including being returned to court.

For a mental health treatment requirement to be made, a Section 12 registered medical practitioner must indicate there is a need for specialist assessment. Recommendation for a mental health treatment requirement must be included within the pre-sentence report, indicating there is a need for it and that there is informed consent from the young person and their parents. The YOS officer needs to ensure that the child or young person is willing to comply with a mental health treatment requirement and be satisfied that they understand what is being proposed and the consequences of any breach.

## Transition

Over 50 per cent of adults with mental health problems were diagnosed in childhood, with less than half of them being treated appropriately at the time (Kim-Cohen et al., 2003). Kessler et al. (2005) showed that half of all lifetime cases of mental illness begin by age 14. These statistics indicate that there is a role for ensuring that young people transition from CAMHS to adult mental health services (AMHS) as smoothly and effectively as possible.

CAMHS is delivered by clinicians with specialist training and experience in working with young people. Some CAMHS practitioners may have had experience and training in AMHS, but often the focus of their professional development will have been with children and young people. Likewise, adult mental health practitioners may have had experience with children and young people but this is much less likely to be the case.

CAMHS and AMHS are commissioned by different teams and have working relationships with different partner agencies. There is significant variation across localities in relation to the transition of care from CAMHS to AMHS. For example, there are different age cut-off points depending on location: some see everyone up to their eighteenth birthday, others stop at 16, while others refer young people as young as 14 to early intervention in psychosis services if they have that type of illness. Still others will only see 16–18-year-olds if they are in full-time education.

Although in adult services carers are considered in the planning of care and assessment of service users, in CAMHS it is a legal requirement for the person with parental responsibility for a young person under 16 to provide consent to assessment and treatment. In addition, the family are seen very much as part of the assessment and care package. As a result of these and other differences, care pathways, protocols, and philosophies of care develop without much collaboration between the CAMHS and adult services.

Moving from CAMHS to AMHS can be a frightening experience for young people. Also, CAMHS tends to have a wider remit than AMHS, with less emphasis on severe mental illnesses, such as psychosis. A study of young people's transitions from CAMHS to AMHS (Singh et al., 2010) found that up to a third of young people are lost from care during transition and a further third experience an interruption in their care. To address this discontinuity of care, local services have started to develop transition services for 16–18-year-olds. Some localities have chosen to expand this to 19-year-olds.

There are many challenges to a smooth transition from CAMHS to AMHS, one of which is that the severity of illness for referral to the service is higher in AMHS than CAMHS. As a result, many young people are left with no support after receiving a comprehensive package of care from CAMHS. The Joint Commissioning Panel for Mental Health (2012) describes how there are five key stages to the transition process for this group of young people:

1. The young person is placed in the 16–19 service.
2. The young person's CAMHS practitioner liaises with the adult mental health service manager to coordinate the transition.
3. A written referral is made, detailing the full mental health assessment details and care plans, and documentation is completed.
4. The adult service confirms, in writing, that they have received the referral and this is copied to other professionals, the young person, and their carer.
5. Clinical responsibility would remain with the 16–19 service if the young person is formally accepted by the adult mental health service. The case file will be transferred with the young person.

Care of young people in transition between CAMHS and adult mental health services should be planned and managed according to the best practice guidance described in the Department of Health's (2006) document, *Transition: Getting it Right for Young People.*

Poor communication between CAMHS and AMHS often leads to repeated assessments, being seen by different clinicians, and different explanations and care plans. The young person's CAMHS practitioner needs to liaise with the AMHS to coordinate the transition, which may involve joint working for a period of time. The written referral to AMHS should involve a full assessment, including risk, history of service involvement, family history, psychopharmacological history, and current care plan.

On receipt of this information, AMHS needs to confirm acceptance of the referral in writing, copying in the relevant professionals, the young person, and their carers. Clinical responsibility remains with CAMHS until formal discharge and acceptance by AMHS. The clinical records should follow the young person and CAMHS should receive a written receipt stating this. In addition, it is important that all agencies that are involved in the care of the young person are involved in the conversations about the transition to AMHS.

## Key messages

- Evidence-based interventions are available in CAMHS. They are continually developing and innovative treatments are emerging.
- A child or young person may benefit from a care or treatment plan that includes a combination of types of intervention.
- One size does not fit all, so it is important to continuously review treatment and adjust it according to the needs of the individual.
- The foundation of all interventions is a good therapeutic relationship.

## Further reading

Micucci, J.A. (2009) *The Adolescent in Family Therapy: Harnessing the Power of Relationships* (2nd edn). New York: Guilford Press.

Preston, J.D., O'Neal, J.H. and Talaga, M.C. (2015) *Child and Adolescent Clinical Psychopharmacology Made Simple* (3rd edn). Oakland, CA: New Harbinger.

Rutter, M. and Taylor, E. (2015) *Child and Adolescent Psychiatry* (6th edn). London: Blackwell.

Stallard, P. (2005) *A Clinician's Guide to Think Good, Feel Good: Using CBT with Children and Young People*. Chichester: Wiley-Blackwell.

# 12 Conclusion

The child and adolescent mental health services, its practices and professionals are deeply immersed in social, cultural, and political contexts. CAMHS is always evolving in response to these ever-changing contexts as well as the evolving evidence base and workforce. Within the context of limited financial resources, CAMHS cannot afford to remain silent, as the needs of the children and young people it is working with need to be heard at local policy and commissioning level.

Financial pressures in local areas may lead commissioners to look for short-term savings, which may have an impact in the longer term. This would likely be through the increased use of in-patient beds and crisis services, resulting in young people not being able to access the services they need in a timely fashion. This will have an impact over the decades to come. CAMHS needs to respond to this and proactively identify ways of preventing problems in the future.

The CAMHS review (DCSF, 2008) reported that services are still fragmented with long waiting lists for treatment and a lack of support when young people are in crisis. What is clear is that when attending to the mental health needs of young people, commitment, input, and investment are required from everyone involved in the delivery of services. Collaborative practices are now seen as the most efficient way of delivering high-quality services and ensuring they are responsive to the needs of children, young people, and their families.

Each locality will have its own unique way of delivering services that has evolved over time, interpreting national policy and addressing local need. This may reflect the professional background of its clinicians or a response to the capacity and capability of the workforce. What is important to bear in mind is that all work conducted by CAMHS is aimed at minimizing the effects of problems that children and young people have while maximizing their developmental potential.

The future of CAMHS holds many opportunities and challenges, and it is likely that it will look very different in the years to come, with services being delivered in alternative venues and through multi-agency partnerships. The skill mix within CAMHS is likely to change in response to an ageing workforce. This, together with fewer professionals being trained in recent years will lead to a shortfall in registered CAMHS practitioners. One way some areas have sought to address this issue is by offering a robust consultation service to schools and primary care, enabling assessment and treatment to take place without the direct involvement of Tier 2 or Tier 3 CAMHS.

*The Five Year Forward View* (NHS England, 2014a) has set the scene for the coming years in health and applies to CAMHS also. It is envisaged that it will involve the NHS but also increasingly it will present services with opportunities to partner with the third sector and private sector to develop new ways of working. *The Five Year Forward View* emphasizes the importance of child health and suggests that 'a radical upgrade in prevention and public health' is needed, although it only relates this to obesity specifically. *The Five Year Forward View* mentions children seven times but only once in relation to mental health. It says:

> We also want to expand access standards to cover a comprehensive range of mental health services, including children's services, eating disorders, and those with bipolar conditions. We need new commissioning approaches to help ensure that happens, and extra staff to coordinate such care. Getting there will require further investment.

With this in mind, CAMHS practitioners will need to be proactive and innovative, focusing on the local population and integrated working with partners such as the third sector, education, social care, and child health.

An emerging area of work with young people, with great potential, is the use of technology. Programmes such as 'Stressbusters' (Wright et al., 2014), an interactive computer software program based on a clinically effective face-to-face CBT protocol for young people with depression, will likely complement face-to-face work. Communication via text, email, and video calls is increasingly being used in services and will become more commonplace as clinicians become more confident in their use and assured of how safe these modes of communication are.

Historically, service user involvement in service design and feedback has usually followed the traditional models used in adult services. When young people are actively involved in co-leading, co-developing, and co-producing services, exciting new services and possibilities arise.

This book has attempted to provide an overview of what CAMHS does, what child and adolescent mental health difficulties are, and how they might be treated. This is a broad brush approach and each area can be explored further by reading the relevant literature. The future of CAMHS, in its current form, may be uncertain but what is certain is that the issue of child and adolescent mental health is not going to go away. More than ever, well-organized services with skilled and caring clinicians will be needed to assist children and young people with mental health problems and their families.

## Key messages

- The future holds many possibilities for integrated working, innovative service design and treatments.
- New roles are likely to be developed in CAMHs as the workforce ages without robust succession planning being in place.
- Service user involvement will likely evolve to include young people in the co-production, co-design, and co-leading of services.

## Further reading

Glasby, J. (2012) *Commissioning for Health and Well-being: An Introduction.* Bristol: Policy Press.

# References

Aldridge, J. and Medina, J. (2008) *Youth Gangs in an English City: Social Exclusion, Drugs and Violence*. Full ESRC End of Award Report, RES-000-23-0615. Swindon: ESRC.

American Psychiatric Association (APA) (2013) *Diagnostic and Statistical Manual of Mental Disorders V*. Washington, DC: APA.

Argyle, M. (1988) *Bodily Communication* (2nd edn). New York: Methuen.

Bailey, S. (1999) The interface between mental health, criminal justice and forensic mental health services for children and adolescents, *Current Opinion in Psychiatry*, 12: 425–32.

Bailey, S. (2002) Violent children: a framework for assessment, *Advances in Psychiatric Treatment*, 8: 97–106.

Bazyk, S. (ed.) (2011) *Mental Health Promotion, Prevention, and Intervention with Children and Youth: A Guiding Framework for Occupational Therapy*. Bethesda, MD: AOTA Press.

Bellman, M., Byrne, O. and Sege, R. (2013) Developmental assessment of children, *British Medical Journal*, 346: e8687.

Berk, L. (2012) *Child Development* 9th (edn). London: Pearson.

Bird, H.B., Yager, T.J., Staghezza, B., Gould, M.S., Canino, G. and Rubio-Stipec, M. (1990) Impairment in the epidemiological measurement of childhood psychopathology in the community, *Journal of the American Academy of Child and Adolescent Psychiatry*, 29: 796–803.

Borum, R., Bartel, P. and Forth, A. (2006) *Structured Assessment for Violence Risk in Youth (SAVRY)*. Tampa, FL: Mental Health Institute, University of South Florida.

Bowlby, J. (1969) *Attachment and Loss, Vol. 1: Attachment*. New York: Basic Books.

British Medical Association and Law Society (1999) *Assessment of Mental Capacity: A Practical Guide for Doctors and Lawyers* (3rd edn) (General editor: P. Letts). Nottingham: Law Society Publishing.

Brotherton, G., Davies, H. and McGillivray, G. (2010) *Working with Children, Young People and Families*. London: Sage.

Butler, R.J. and Heron, J. (2008) The prevalence of infrequent bedwetting and nocturnal enuresis in childhood: a large British cohort, *Scandinavian Journal of Urology and Nephrology*, 42: 257–64.

Caspi, A., McClay, J., Moffitt, T.E., Mill, J., Martin, J. and Craig, I.W. (2002) Role of genotype in the cycle of violence in maltreated children, *Science*, 297: 851–4.

Crown (1958) *Public Records Act*. London: HMSO.

Crown (1969) *Family Reform Act*. London: HMSO.

Crown (1983) *Mental Health Act*. London: HMSO.

Crown (1987) *Family Reform Act*. London: HMSO.

Crown (1989) *Children Act*. London: HMSO.

Crown (1998) *Crime and Disorder Act*. London: HMSO.

Crown (2004) *Children Act*. Norwich: HMSO.

Crown (2005) *Mental Capacity Act*. London: The Stationery Office.

Crown (2007) *Mental Health Act*. London: HMSO.

Davis, H. and Day, C. (2010) *Working in Partnership with Parents* (2nd edn). London: Pearson.

Day, C., Ellis, M. and Harris, L. (2015) *The Family Partnership Model Reflective Practice Handbook*. London: The Centre for Parent and Child Support.

Department for Children, Schools and Families (DCSF) (2007) *The Children's Plan: Building Brighter Futures*. London: The Stationery Office.

Department for Children, Schools and Families (DCSF) (2008) *Children and Young People in Mind*. Final Report of the National CAMHS Review. Nottingham: DCSF Publications.

Department for Children, Schools and Families/Department of Health (DCSF/DoH) (2010) *Keeping Children and Young People in Mind: The Government's Full Response to the Independent Review of CAMHS*. Nottingham: DCSF Publications.

Department for Education (DfE) (2011) *Me and My School: Findings from the National Evaluation of Targeted Mental Health in Schools 2008–2011*. London: Department of Health.

Department for Education (DfE) (2012) *Positive for Youth: A New Approach to Cross-Government Policy for Young People Aged 13 to 19*. London: DfE.

Department for Education and Skills (DfES) (2003) *Every Child Matters*. Nottingham: DfES Publications.

Department of Health (1995) *Together We Stand: Commissioning, Role and Management of Child and Adolescent Mental Health Services* (NHS Health Advisory Service Thematic Reviews). London: Department of Health.

Department of Health (1998) *Quality Protects*. London: Department of Health.

Department of Health (1999) *Clinical Governance in the New NHS*. London: Department of Health.

Department of Health (2000) *The NHS Plan Implementation Programme*. London: Department of Health.

Department of Health (2003) *The National Service Framework*. London: Department of Health.

Department of Health (2006) *Transition: Getting it Right for Young People*. London: Department of Health.

Department of Health (2009) *New Horizons: A Shared Vision for Mental Health*. London: Department of Health.

Department of Health (2011a) *No Health without Mental Health: A Cross-Government Mental Health Outcomes Strategy for People of All Ages*. London: Department of Health.

Department of Health (2011b) *Talking Therapies: A Four-Year Plan of Action*. London: Department of Health.

Dew, M.A., Dunn, L.O., Bromet, E.J. and Schulberg, H.C. (1998) Factors affecting help-seeking during depression in a community sample, *Journal of Affective Disorders*, 14: 223–34.

Dolan, M., Holloway, J., Bailey, S. and Smith, C. (1999) Health status of juvenile offenders: a survey of young offenders appearing before the juvenile courts, *Journal of Adolescence*, 22: 137–44.

Dwivedi, K.N. (2004) *Promoting the Emotional Well-Being of Children and Adolescents and Preventing Their Mental Ill Health: A Handbook*. London: Jessica Kingsley.

Esbensen, F.-A. and Weerman, F. (2005) Youth gangs and troublesome youth groups in the United States and the Netherlands: a cross-national comparison, *European Journal of Criminology*, 2: 5–37.

Fernando, S. (1991) *Mental Health, Race and Culture*. London: Mind Publications.

Foley, D.L., Eaves, L.J., Wormley, B., Silberg, J.L., Maes, H.H., Kuhn, J. et al. (2004) Childhood adversity, monoamine oxidase A genotype, and risk for conduct disorder, *Archives of General Psychiatry*, 61: 738–44.

Geldard, K. (2009) *Practical Interventions for Young People at Risk*. London: Sage.

Gilvarry, E., McArdle, P., O'Herlihy, A., Mirza, K.A.H., Bevington, D. and Malcolm, N.

(2012) *Practice Standards for Young People with Substance Misuse Problems.* London: Royal College of Psychiatrists.

Glasby, J. (2012) *Commissioning for Health and Well-being: An Introduction.* Bristol: Policy Press.

Glenny, G. and Roaf, C. (2008) *Multiprofessional Communication: Making Systems Work for Children.* Maidenhead: Open University Press.

Goodman, R. (1997) The Strengths and Difficulties Questionnaire: a research note, *Journal of Child Psychology and Psychiatry,* 38: 581–6.

Goodman, R., Ford, T., Simmon, H., Gatward, R. and Meltzer, H. (2000) Using the Strengths and Difficulties Questionnaire (SDQ) to screen for child psychiatric disorders in a community sample, *British Journal of Psychiatry,* 177: 534–9.

Goodman, R. and Scott, S. (2012) *Child and Adolescent Psychiatry* (3rd edn.). Chichester: Wiley-Blackwell.

Green, H., Mcginnity, A., Meltzer, H., Ford, T. and Goodman, R. (2005) *Mental Health of Children and Adolescents in Great Britain 2004.* London: ONS.

Harper, R. (2014) *Medical Treatment and the Law: Issues of Consent. The Protection of the Vulnerable: Children and Adults Lacking Capacity* (2nd edn). Bristol: Family Law.

Hodes, M. (2000) Psychologically distressed refugee children in the United Kingdom, *Child Psychology and Psychiatry Review,* 5: 57–68.

James, A.C., Taylor, A., Winmill, L. and Alfoadari, K. (2008) A preliminary community study of dialectical behaviour therapy (DBT) with adolescent females demonstrating persistent, deliberate self-harm (DSH), *Child and Adolescent Mental Health,* 13: 148–52.

Joint Commissioning Panel for Mental Health (2012) *Guidance for Commissioners of Mental Health Services for Young People Making the Transition from Child and Adolescent to Adult Services, Vol. 2: Practical Mental Health commissioning* [http://www.rcpsych. ac.uk/PDF/JCP-MH%20CAMHS%20transitions%20(March%202012).pdf].

Jorm, A.F. (2000) Mental health literacy: public knowledge and beliefs about mental disorders, *British Journal of Psychiatry,* 177: 396–401.

Jorm, A.F., Korten, A.E. and Jacomb, P.A. (1997) Helpfulness of interventions for mental disorders: beliefs of health professionals compared with the general public, *British Journal of Psychiatry,* 171: 233–7.

Kalid, K. (2013) *A Practical Guide to Mental Health Problems in Children with Autistic Spectrum: It's Not Just Their Autism!* London: Jessica Kingsley.

Kessler, R.C., Chiu, W.T., Demler, O., Merikangas, K.R. and Walters, E.E. (2005) Prevalence, severity, and comorbidity of 12-month DSM-IV disorders in the National Comorbidity Survey Replication, *Archives of General Psychiatry,* 62: 617–27.

Kim-Cohen, J., Caspi, A., Moffitt, T.E., Harrington, H., Milne, B.J. and Poulton, R. (2003) Prior juvenile diagnoses in adults with mental disorder, *Archives of General Psychiatry,* 60: 709–17.

Kim-Cohen, J., Caspi, A., Taylor, A., Williams, B., Newcombe, R. and Craig, I.W. (2006) Maltreatment, and gene–environment interactions predicting children's mental health: new evidence and a meta-analysis, *Molecular Psychiatry,* 11: 903–13.

Krausz, M., Müller-Thomsen, T. and Haasen, C. (1995) Suicide among schizophrenic adolescents in the long-term course of illness, *Psychopathology,* 28: 95–103.

Kurtz, Z., Thornes, R. and Wolkind, S. (1994) *Services for the Mental Health of Children and Young People in England: A National Review.* London: Maudsley Hospital and South Thames (West) Regional Health Authority.

Laming, H. (2003) *The Victoria Climbié Inquiry.* Report of an Inquiry by Lord Laming. London: The Stationery Office.

Lask, B. and Bryant-Waugh, R. (eds) (2013) *Eating Disorders in Childhood and Adolescence*. London: Routledge.

Lay, B., Blanz, B., Hartmann, M. and Schmidt, M.H. (2000) The psychosocial outcome of adolescent-onset schizophrenia: a 12-year followup, *Schizophrenia Bulletin*, 26: 801–16.

Lipsedge, M. and Littlewood, R. (1997) *Aliens and Alienists: Ethnic Minorities and Psychiatry* (3rd edn). London: Routledge.

Loeber, R., Burke, J.D. and Lahey, B.B. (2002) What are adolescent antecedents to antisocial personality disorder?, *Criminal Behaviour and Mental Health*, 12(1): 24–36.

Mental Health Foundation (MHF) (1999) *A Bright Future for All: Promoting Mental Health in Education*. London: MHF.

Micucci, J.A. (2009) *The Adolescent in Family Therapy: Harnessing the Power of Relationships* (2nd edn). New York: Guilford Press.

Mordre, M., Groholt, B., Kjelsberg, E., Sandstad, B. and Myhre, A.M. (2011) The impact of ADHD and conduct disorder in childhood on adult delinquency: a 30 years follow-up study using official crime records, *BMC Psychiatry*, 11: 57.

National Collaborating Centre for Mental Health (NCCMH) (2014) E-therapies Systematic Review for Children and Young People with Mental Health Problems [https://www.minded.org.uk/pluginfile.php/1287/course/section/579/e-Therapies%20link2%20-%20Full%20Review%20-%20v0.2%2021.3.14.pdf].

NHS England (2014a) *The Five Year Forward View* [http://www.england.nhs.uk/wp-content/uploads/2014/10/5yfv-web.pdf].

NHS England (2014b) *Child and Adolescent Mental Health Services (CAMHS) Tier 4 Report* [http://www.england.nhs.uk/wp-content/uploads/2014/07/camhs-tier-4-rep.pdf].

NICE (2004a) *Eating Disorders* (CG9). London: NICE [http://www.nice.org.uk/guidance].

NICE (2004b) *Self-harm* (CG16). London: NICE [http://www.nice.org.uk/guidance].

NICE (2005a) *Obsessive-Compulsive Disorder* (CG31). London: NICE [http://www.nice.org.uk/guidance].

NICE (2005b) *Post-Traumatic Stress Disorder (PTSD): The Management of PTSD in Adults and Children in Primary and Secondary Care* (CG26). London: NICE [http://www.nice.org.uk/guidance].

NICE (2005c) *Depression in Children and Young People: Identification and Management in Primary, Community and Secondary Care* (CG28). London: NICE [http://www.nice.org.uk/guidance/cg28].

NICE (2007) *Urinary Tract Infection in Children* (CG54). London: NICE [http://www.nice.org.uk/guidance].

NICE (2008a) *Social and Emotional Wellbeing for Children and Young People in Primary School* (PH12). London: NICE [http://www.nice.org.uk/guidance].

NICE (2008b) *Attention Deficit Hyperactivity Disorder: Diagnosis and Management of ADHD in Children, Young People and Adults*. London: NICE [http://www.nice.org.uk/guidance].

NICE (2009a) *Coeliac Disease* (CG86). London: NICE [http://www.nice.org.uk/guidance].

NICE (2009b) *Social and Emotional Wellbeing for Children and Young People in Secondary School* (PH20). London: NICE [http://www.nice.org.uk/guidance].

NICE (2009c) *When to Suspect Child Maltreatment* (CG89). London: NICE [http://www.nice.org.uk/guidance].

NICE (2010a) *Constipation in Children and Young People: Diagnosis and Management of Idiopathic Childhood Constipation in Primary and Secondary Care* (CG99). London: NICE [http://www.nice.org.uk/guidance].

NICE (2010b) *Nocturnal Enuresis* (CG111). London: NICE [http://www.nice.org.uk/guidance].

NICE (2011) *Self-harm: Longer-term Management* (CG133). London: NICE [http://www.nice.org.uk/guidance].

NICE (2013a) *Antisocial Behaviour and Conduct Disorders in Children and Young People: Recognition, Intervention and Management* (CG158). London: NICE [http://www.nice.org.uk/guidance].

NICE (2013b) *Psychosis and Schizophrenia in Children and Young People: Recognition and Management* (CG155). London: NICE [http://www.nice.org.uk/guidance].

NICE (2013c) *Quality Standard for Self-harm* (QS34). London: NICE [http://www.nice.org.uk/guidance].

NICE (2014) *Treatment Occurring in Paediatrics (STOP): Assessing and Monitoring Risk of Suicide in Children and Adolescents.* London: NICE [http://www.nice.org.uk/guidance].

Nutbeam, D., Wise, M., Bauman, A., Harris, E. and Leeder, S. (1993) *Goals and Targets for Australia's Health in the Year 2000 and Beyond.* Canberra, ACT: Australian Government Publishing Service.

Olsson, C.A., Bond, L., Burns, J.M., Vella-Brodrick, D.A. and Sawyer, S.M. (2003) Adolescent resilience: a concept analysis, *Journal of Adolescence*, 26: 1–11.

Pearce, C. (2011) *A Short Introduction to Promoting Resilience in Children* (JKP Short Introductions). London: Jessica Kingsley.

Powell, C. (2011) *Safeguarding and Child Protection for Nurses, Midwives and Health Visitors: A Practical Guide.* Maidenhead: Open University Press.

Preston, J.D., O'Neal, J.H. and Talaga, M.C. (2015) *Child and Adolescent Clinical Psychopharmacology Made Simple* (3rd edn.). Oakland, CA: New Harbinger.

Rutter, M. and Taylor, E. (2015) *Child and Adolescent Psychiatry* (6th edn). London: Blackwell.

Satterfield, J.H., Faller, K.J., Crinella, F.M., Schell, A., Swanson, J.M. and Homer, L.D. (2007) A 30-year prospective follow-up study of hyperactive boys with conduct problems: adult criminality, *Journal of the American Academy of Child and Adolescent Psychiatry*, 46: 601–10.

Scarman, L.G. (1985) *Gillick v West Norfolk and Wisbech Area Health Authority and another* [http://cirp.org/library/legal/UKlaw/gillickvwestnorfolk1985/].

Singh, S.P., Moli, P., Ford, T., Kramer, T., McLaren, S. and Hovish, K. (2010) Process, outcome and experience of transition from child to adult mental healthcare: multiperspective study, *British Journal of Psychiatry*, 197: 305–12.

Stallard, P. (2005) *A Clinician's Guide to Think Good, Feel Good: Using CBT with Children and Young People.* Chichester: Wiley-Blackwell.

Teplin, L.A., Abram, K.M., McCelland, G.M., Dulcan, M.K. and Mericle, A.A. (2002) Psychiatric disorders in youth in juvenile detention, *Archives of General Psychiatry*, 59: 1133–43.

UN General Assembly (1989) *Convention on the Rights of the Child.* UN Treaty Series, 1577, 3. New York: United Nations.

Weerman, F.M., Maxson, C.L., Esbensen, F.A., Aldridge, J., Medina, J. and Van Gemert, F. (2009) *Eurogang Program Manual: Background, Development and Use of the Eurogang Instruments in Multi-site, Multi-method Comparative Research* [www.umsl.edu/ccj/Eurogang/EurogangManual.pdf].

Weinstein, D., Staffelbach, D. and Biaggio, M. (2000) Attention-deficit hyperactivity disorder and posttraumatic stress disorder: differential diagnosis in childhood sexual abuse, *Clinical Psychology Review*, 20: 359–78.

White, M (1968) *Beating Sneaky Poo* [http://www.narrativetherapylibrary.com/media/downloadable/files/links/b/e/beating-sneaky-poo-2_2.pdf].

Williams, R. and Keerfoot, M. (2005) *Child and Adolescent Mental Health Services: Strategy, Planning, Delivery, and Evaluation.* Oxford: Oxford University Press.

World Health Organization (WHO) (1992) *The ICD-10 Classification of Mental and Behavioural Disorders.* Geneva: WHO.

World Health Organization (WHO) (1996) *Multiaxial Classification of Child and Adolescent Psychiatric Disorders: The ICD-10 Classification of Mental and Behavioural Disorders in Children and Adolescents.* Cambridge: Cambridge University Press.

Worling, J.R. (2013) *Desistence for Adolescents who Sexually Harm (DASH-13)* [http://www.erasor.org/new-protective-factors.html].

Worling, J.R. and Curwen, T. (2001) Estimate of Risk of Adolescent Sexual Offense Recidivism (Version 2.0: The "ERASOR"), in M.C. Calder (ed.) *Juveniles and Children Who Sexually Abuse: Frameworks for Assessment* (pp. 372–97). Lyme Regis: Russell House Publishing.

Wright, B., Tindall, L., Littlewood, E., Adamson, J., Allgar, V, Bennett, S. et al. (2014) Computerised cognitive behaviour therapy for depression in adolescents: study protocol for a feasibility randomised controlled trial, *British Medical Journal Open* [http://www.researchgate.net/publication/267745766_Computerised_cognitive_behaviour_therapy_for_depression_in_adolescents_study_protocol_for_a_feasibility_randomised_controlled_trial].

Wrycraft, N. (2015) Partnership working, in *Assessment and Care Planning in Mental Health Nursing.* Maidenhead: Open University Press.

Yehuda, R. (2001) Biology of posttraumatic stress disorder, *Journal of Clinical Psychiatry*, 62: 41–6.

Youth Justice Board for England and Wales (2011) *SIFA and SQIFA* [https://www.gov.uk/government/publications/young-offenders-assessment-using-sifa-and-sqifa].

# Web resources

| Organization | Subject | Website |
| --- | --- | --- |
| Anxiety UK | Anxiety | www.anxietyuk.org.uk |
| Bipolar UK | Bipolar affective disorder | www.bipolaruk.org.uk |
| The Centre for Parent and Child Support | The Family Partnership Model, Empowering Parents, Empowering Communities and the Helping Families Programme | www.cpcs.org.uk |
| Childline | Child support | https://www.childline.org.uk |
| Children and Young People's Improving Access to Psychological Therapies (CYP-IAPT) | CYP-IAPT | www.cypiapt.org. |
| Choice and Partnership Approach (CAPA) | Service organization | www.camhsnetwork.co.uk |
| Child Outcomes Research Consortium (CORC) | Outcome measures | www.corc.uk.net |
| ERIC | Enuresis and encopresis | www.eric.org.uk |
| Minded | All child and adolescent mental health issues | www.minded.org.uk |
| National ADD Information and Support Service (ADDISS) | ADHD | www.addiss.co.uk |
| The National Autistic Society | Autism and Asperger's | www.autism.org.uk |
| OCD-UK | Obsessive-compulsive disorder | www.ocduk.org |
| Royal College of Psychiatrists | All child and adolescent mental health issues | http://www.rcpsych.ac.uk/expertadvice/youthinfo |
| UK ADHD Partnership (UKAP) | ADHD | www.ukadhd.org |
| Youngminds | All child and adolescent mental health issues | www.youngminds.org.uk |

# Index

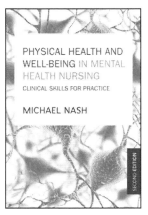

**PHYSICAL HEALTH AND WELL-BEING IN MENTAL HEALTH NURSING**
Clinical Skills for Practice
Second Edition

Michael Nash

ISBN: 9780335262861 (Paperback)
ebook: 9780335262878
2014

This popular and groundbreaking book was the first of its kind to focus on providing mental health nurses with the core knowledge of the physical health issues that they need for their work. Considering the risk factors and assessment priorities amongst different mental health client groups, the book provides clinical insights and current guidance into how best to work with service users to ensure their health is assessed and improved.

In this fully updated second edition the book addresses the current context and the latest research and policy, as well as expanding coverage of:

- Assessment principles and skills
- Adverse reactions, side effects and service user and family education
- Working with older and younger service users
- Multi-professional working

www.openup.co.uk

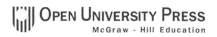

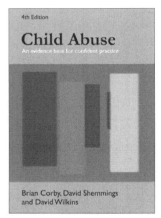

## CHILD ABUSE
An Evidence Base for Confident Practice
Fourth Edition

Brian Corby, David Shemmings and David Wilkins

ISBN: 9780335245093 (Paperback)
ebook: 9780335245109
2012

This best-selling text has been used by countless students, practitioners and researchers as a key reference on child protection issues. The book demystifies this complex and emotionally-charged area, outlining research, history, social policy and legislation, as well as the theory and practice underpinning child protection work.

**Key features:**

- The latest research and thinking on the causes of child abuse, including new insights from the field of attachment theory
- An updated overview of child protection practices, ranging from the 19th Century to the recent 'Baby P' tragedy
- Detailed analysis and coverage of the Munro review of child protection in England and the work of the Social Work Reform Board

www.openup.co.uk

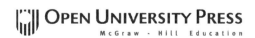

OPEN UNIVERSITY PRESS
McGraw - Hill Education